Own Your Health: Ayurveda for Everyone

Verses Kindler Publication.

Verses Kindler Publication.

Website: www.verseskindlerpublication.com

Own Your Health:Ayurveda for Everyone

By: Dr. Soumya Kashi

ISBN: 978-93-49532-43-4

NON-FICTION STORIES 1st Edition

Price: INR 399/$20

Disclaimer

Own Your Health: Ayurveda for Everyone is written by Dr. Soumya Kashi.

The published work is the original contents of the author and she has done her best to edit and make it error-free.

The opinions/ contents expressed in this book are solely of the author and do not represent the opinions/ standings/ thoughts of the publisher. Any resemblance of names of actual person, place or institute is purely coincidental to carry forward the story.

The write-up is the original content of the author and the author is solely responsible for it, the publisher would not be responsible for it.

Index

Table of Contents

Introduction: A Journey into the Heart of Ayurveda

Ayurveda is the ancient science of life that has guided human beings throughout the ages. This book bridges the gap between its ancient principles and modern living. Ayurveda provides a roadmap to rediscovering harmony, vitality, and purpose in this modern world of pressure, disease, and imbalances. It is a full-fledged compendium explaining the basic premises of Ayurveda and its practical and profound capacity to influence health and well-being.

Who is This Book For?

This book is for everyone, not only those familiar with the Ayurvedic tradition but also those who want to learn about Ayurveda more closely to meet their needs. It will be a helpful resource for busy professionals and curious seekers seeking ways to improve their well-being or practitioners who want to use practical insights. Consider these teachings and perceive the body, mind, and spirit differently while taking practical steps toward living in balanced harmony.

What Does This Book Have In Store For You?

This is an exquisite tapestry of Ayurvedic wisdom with ancient principles interwoven and practical applications that start off introducing us to the foundational concepts of Ayurveda that include Tridoshas or the three core types of energies-Vata, Pitta, and

Kapha: Agni or digestive fire; and Prakriti or constitution-by defining how these factors shape our overall health and well-being.

From there, it moves into the practical tools of daily living, including routines called Dinacharya and seasonal adjustments known as Ritucharya, all the way to the rhythms of nature. There, readers will learn about Panchakarma therapies, robust detoxification processes that cleanse and rejuvenate the body, and the role of herbal remedies and dietary practices tailored to the individual.

Emphasis has been placed on the mind-body relationship, and Shirodhara and Nasya therapies have been discussed, which soothe the mind and bring clarity. Besides, Yoga and pranayama as complementary practices that bring harmony to the physical and mental aspects of health have been discussed.

Based on two decades of my experience practicing Ayurveda, I explain how ancient Ayurvedic principles can surmount such modern challenges with the help of case stories, stories, and real-life applications to stress, chronic ailments, and lifestyle diseases. The final chapters combine it with step-by-step actions to incorporate Ayurveda into everyday life.

How Does This Book Help?

This book makes Ayurveda relevant to life and accessible to everyone. It demystifies this ancient science and shows it as a practical, holistic approach to health and wellness. The book puts the reader in charge of their well-being and gives them the tools to prevent disease, restore balance, and cultivate vitality. By the end of this book, you'll know Ayurveda and be empowered to live it. I recommend that you follow the knowledge of this book under the guidance of an Ayurveda doctor.

Chapter 1: The Essence of Ayurveda

- **The Soul of it all**

A long time ago, kings and kingdoms thrived without the facilities and luxuries we enjoy. Even more robust and healthier than us, our ancestors followed a way of living that helped them prosper and nourish. Yes, you have guessed it right. Ayurveda - commonly and aptly called the "Science of Life," is a categorically ancient medical system, but indeed, a deep, compelling philosophy of life that has stood the test of time. Imagine wisdom so timeless and intrinsic that it emerged at the very beginning of creation itself.

It is believed that Ayurveda emerged from the churning cosmic ocean, where gods and demons sought the elixir of immortality. As it were, Ayurveda emerged from the bottom of the sea as a gift from the gods—a clue to nature about the appropriate way of maintaining balance and harmony in life. The sage Atreya then gave it to humanity, teaching this holy wisdom to his students.

- **History's Treasure**

Ayurveda originated in ancient Indian culture, and its texts, including the Charaka Samhita and the Sushruta Samhita, were written over 5,000 years ago. These texts are not medical texts but scriptures harmoniously relating to nature. They speak to a time when sages observed the natural world and realized that the secrets to human health were contained therein. The sages saw how the five elements of earth, water, fire, air, and space combined and transformed into the human body.

This means that Ayurveda is not strictly a medicine in the classical sense but a complete life system and culture that acknowledges the intrinsic connection linking all its various parts and facets.

- **The Pillar-Principles of Ayurveda**

Balance is a relatively simple yet profound premise at the very heart of Ayurveda. The human body is an intricate balance of three doshas, or humours - Vata, Pitta, and Kapha- relating to natural elements: the senses, mind, and soul. Vata, or the energy of movement, can be linked to air and space; Pitta, or the energy of transformation, is related to fire and water; Kapha, or structure and lubrication, is related to earth and water. To achieve life's purposes, one needs to balance one's doshas, senses, mind, and soul because diseases diminish a nourishing and healthy life.

Think about this: if we are feeling "off," it's often because something is out of balance. We have been having too much spicy food, and our Pitta has become aggravated, leading to acidity or irritability; or maybe we have been being too passive, which causes our Kapha to increase, leading us to become sluggish and gain weight. Ayurveda teaches the healthy and those suffering from diseases to recognize these signs and adjust their lifestyles appropriately, like tuning a musical instrument to keep it in perfect harmony.

Ayurveda teaches the principle of "like increases like and opposite balance." If you feel hot and fiery or have excess Pitta, eat cooling foods such as cucumber and coconut water to find balance. Conversely, warming spices such as ginger and black pepper can help rekindle your inner heat if you feel cold and sluggish or have excess Kapha.

Approaches to Holistic Health and Wellness

Ayurveda seeks more than symptom management; it seeks the root of any imbalance. This way of life teaches harmony with nature and one's inner self. Ayurveda confirms that health is the absence of disease and a condition of harmonious physical, mental, and social well-being.

The term "Ayu" is the conjunction of the body with the senses, mind, and soul.

We must be healthy on all these levels to lead healthy lives, fulfill our obligations, enjoy life, create wealth, and ultimately work toward salvation. Ayurveda provides the means of acquiring this integrated health, with its therapeutic philosophy emphasizing both disease prevention and health promotion.

Take the story of Asha, age 45, who had a good job, family, and friends. She was living as a tired, irritable person who was always unfulfilled. She came to Ayurveda for help with more than her chronic headaches and indigestion but also to understand why she felt so disconnected. Through Ayurvedic guidance, Asha learned to align her daily routines, called *Dincharya*, with seasonal practices, called *Ritucharya*, based on nature's rhythms. She followed a diet according to her dosha and did conscious breathing, and slowly, her headaches and gastrointestinal problems started to disappear. More importantly, she found new meaning and involvement in life. Indeed, Asha is a perfect example of Ayurveda's comprehensive approach to body, mind, and spirit to achieve healthy well-being.

Ayurveda, fundamentally, is the art of maintaining awareness of life processes. It sees life as a divine journey and teaches that our health and well-being are inextricably linked to everything around us: the foods we eat, the thoughts we think, the air we breathe, and the actions we take.

Ayurveda considers the human individual a microcosm of the universe, consisting of the same five elements: air, space, fire, water, and earth. Apart from these elements, Ayurveda then acknowledges the soul, mind, time, and direction as forming, together with the earlier ten nine components influencing our health. These have to be in balance within us as they have to be in balance in the universe. Diseases manifest when this balance is disturbed by overuse, underuse, or abuse of time, senses, or intelligence. For example, too much sunfire can lead to heatstroke, while too much cold food can diminish the digestive fire and cause indigestion. Ayurveda supports us in regaining this balance and, henceforth, bringing harmony and well-being.

Apart from this, Ayurveda teaches that diseases don't just happen. They result from imbalance, be it from an unusual climate, inappropriate food choices, or negative thoughts. For instance, Ramesh had been working a very stressful job for a long time and was attracted to junk food and late-night binge-watching, further aggravating his imbalances. Only after listening to his body did he make conscious changes in his lifestyle: he began to choose nourishing foods, practiced relaxation techniques, and welcomed positivity into his life.

As is clear now, Ayurveda is not some general panacea; it is an individualized scientific consideration of one's unique constitutional and life circumstances. Instead, it allows us to take responsibility for our health and be more aware of our bodies while ensuring that our unique needs are understood and catered for. Ayurveda teaches us to live harmoniously with the surrounding environment, promoting balance and well-being.

- **To sum it all up:**

Ayurveda provides a path to living long and well. Embracing its precepts means learning to listen to our bodies, respect our minds, and nourish our souls. We realize that health is not a destination but a journey—a dance with nature's rhythms and our inner selves. In a world that feels disconnected and out of sync, Ayurveda returns the map to balance, harmony, and well-being.

As we embark on this journey together, remember that Ayurveda is other than remedies or treatments; it is a life lived to honor the very existence itself. It's a call back to the core of who we are, to live each day with awareness, gratitude, and joy.

Chapter 2: The Triplet of Equilibrium - Vata, Pitta, Kapha

- **Understanding Tridoshas**

Imagine: There have been days when you feel light and airy, breezing through your workday like summer air. Then there were the days when you just clicked into it, and all of your problems disappeared with the touch of a thought- or vice versa. On those days, you felt pointed to the middle, calm, cool, and collected. Ups and downs in feeling are not an accident but reflect the equipoise of the three doshas, namely Vata, Pitta, and Kapha.

In the Ayurveda tradition, these three doshas represent the prime motor forces behind everything in conjunction with body and mind. Each dosha is derived from five elements: earth, water, fire, air, and space. Each shows how those elements come together and manifest themselves inside us. Tuning the doshas is fine-tuning a guitar to play its best melody for vibrant health and well-being.

Each of us has a dosha constitution, or predominance of Vata, Pitta, and Kapha peculiar to each individual, with its peculiar characteristics determining our physical, mental, and emotional trends blueprint uniquely ours, which defines our natural state. However, according to our lifestyle, diet, or environment, if any of these doshas get imbalanced, we start feeling that in the form of symptoms in body and mind.

- **Functions of Vata, Pitta, and Kapha**

Let us look at the individual doshas, which are central to sustaining balance and health.

- **Vata: The Energy of Motion**

The movement of Vata is responsible for the bodily and mental motions. Think about a gust of wind passing through the trees- that's Vata in motion. It incorporates air and space with lightness, roughness, dryness, and speed.

All movements, from the rising and falling motion of the chest with every breath to the flow of blood, govern the contraction of the muscles and the flow of blood—even the blinking of the eyes. In the mind, Vata is the source of curiosity and mental agility. Each dhatu type has its responsibility, like the prana type, which brings intelligence; speech is the role of udana; and vyana takes care of heart health.

Vata's characteristic physical properties are dry, cold, light, tiny, active, and rough. Foods and herbs that are lubricating, warm, stable, heavy, unctuous, and oily help stabilize Vata's imbalance.

When balanced, vata makes you feel enthusiastic, lively, and adaptable. An imbalance of Vata acts like a storm that has blown in: You may feel anxious, scattered, or restless; your body may become dry, bloated, or fatigued.

Think of the last time you overdid it, doing too many things at once and consequently feeling overwhelmed or frazzled—a classic sign of

Vata imbalance. To balance Vata, you must implement grounding in yoga, warm, nourishing foods, and a stable daily routine.

- **Pitta: The Energy of Transformation**

Thank Pitta if you ever win prizes for a razor-sharp brain or willpower. Pitta is a fire-water dosha that governs digestion and metabolism and produces energy. That power transmutes food into nutrients and ideas into practice. Heat, sharpness, and intensity set Pitta apart as the driving force behind ambition and determination.

Pitta Properties include lubricating, liquidy, warm, pungent, sour, and bitter. Each type of pitta plays a key role in our body. For example, the pachak type brings warmth and initiates metabolism, the bhajan brings a complexion, and the sadhak type brings ego and wisdom.

Pitta digests food, absorbs nutrients, and maintains the body's proper temperature. It also fuels our intellect and lends us clarity and focus. Foods and herbs that are cold, soft, stable, sweet, and astringent will stabilize Pitta imbalances.

When in balance, Pitta keeps us motivated, disciplined, and clear-headed. But when Pitta gets too overboard, you know what happens when fire gets too hot, don't you? You may feel irritated, impatient, or overwhelmingly critical. Physically, you may develop acidity, rashes on your skin, or inflammation.

Do you remember that friend who always dives head-on into whatever challenge he faces and starts to steam when things aren't going exactly his way? That is Pitta, all fired up. To douse it, Pitta needs soothing activities: meditation, cooling foods, a walk in the moonlight, and getaways into nature.

- **Kapha: The Energy of Structure and Stability**

Kapha is structure, lubrication, and stability in body and mind. The heaviness of kapha, its stability, and its nourishing effect come from its earth and water composition- limestone rock, the stability of your mountain, or the serene feeling of your body after a deep sleep. Kapha Properties are- heavy, cold, soft, lubricating, sweet, stable, and slimy. Each kapha type has a unique responsibility; for instance, the book type allows us to recognize taste, and tarpak brings calmness to the brain and senses.

Kapha controls body tissues such as muscles, bones, and fat. It keeps joints moist and moving smoothly and maintains healthy skin. It cools the nervous system and brings peace, patience, and emotional stability. Foods and herbs that stabilize Kapha's imbalance are light, warm, hard, dry, bitter, unstable, and rough.

When balanced, Kapha makes a person feel stable, compassionate, and level-headed. When Kapha is excessive, it makes a person lazy, lethargic, and fearful of change. Maybe you've emerged from the storm heavier, clogged up, or clung to your ritualistic comfort habits.

And who doesn't have that one rock of a person in their lives—predictable, never riled, and cool as a cucumber when the chips are down? Kapha energy works in all the best ways. If there's too much Kapha, energizing, stimulating activities such as exercise, spicy foods, and new experiences will balance it.

- **Dosha Seats and Their Significance**

Let's assume that all the doshas have key spots in the body where their energy may be most concentrated. These principal spots are essential because they provide clues about where imbalances might occur. Knowledge of such centers will help us maintain good health by targeting the right place for healing.

Vata is mainly located in the large intestine/colon, waist, and legs and is responsible for being present and flowing freely throughout the body. Its subsidiary sites are bones, joints, and ears. Vata's disharmony relates to constipation, arthritis, and dry skin conditions.

Pitta is responsible for digestion and metabolism and is found in the navel, stomach, small intestine, sweat and lymph glands, vascular tissue, and circulatory system. It is also subordinate to the eyes, blood, and skin. An imbalance of the dosha can result in heartburn, skin rashes, or problems with vision.

Kapha residences are in the lungs, chest, throat, vascular tissue, fatty tissue, and lungs. Kapha controls the amount of mucus and fluids finding a place within the body. An excess Kapha can thus be held responsible for problems in breathing, congestion, and extra pounds.

Think of them as checkpoints: when something starts to go wrong, you know where to look for the dosha's seat— where the imbalance originates and how to correct it.

- **Dosha Maintenance for Health**

Proper health and wellness arise from balance among Vata, Pitta, and Kapha. According to Ayurveda, when the doshas are in good alignment, a person is no longer just in good physical shape but clearly mentally and emotionally complete. Now, it's just not going to happen in real life that things such as stress, diet, weather-even the seasons-are pushing our doshas off-center. Happily, that is not a problem because Ayurveda hands us the tools to bring them back into balance.

Just think of how jumpy it would be to get up in the morning feeling on edge, one's mind racing a hundred miles an hour. That would be a clue that your Vata is off-kilter. Ayurveda suggests slowing down your activities, eating more warming foods like soups or stews, and focusing on breathing to dampen this storm brewing inside.

You may have already started to feel irritable and cranky about everything. You find yourself yelling at the family; your stomach turns into a crucible of acid. That is the fire of irritated Pitta. You can cool the fire inside of you. They turn to foods like cucumber and coconut water or herbs like mint. They emerge from situations of stress, and the time they have to spend outdoors cools the flames.

When the body feels heavy and you have no energy to mobilize, Kapha sneaks up on you. According to Ayurveda, we should shake off that extra by getting active: take a brisk walk, spice up your meal with some spice, and break loose from stagnating routines that may hold one hostage.

It describes how Ayurveda defines health maintenance as treatment directed toward symptoms and healing the root of any imbalance. Finally, it trains us to learn how to listen to our bodies and takes proactive steps in nurturing our doshas toward living vibrant and balanced lives.

- **To Conclude:**

Ayurveda sees the path to health as an exquisite dance with the doshas, learning how they are in and out of rhythm. By deepening one's knowledge about the Vata, Pitta, and Kapha and regarding the role each of these doshas plays in our well-being, one can devise a way of living that nourishes balance and vitality. With that in mind, we can look after the body and mind in ways that cultivate a life of lasting health, happiness, and peace of mind.

Chapter 3: Ayurvedic Constitution of Body and Type

- **Prakriti or Concept of Body Constitution**

Imagine a room filled with people- some wiry and thin, others slow and sluggish. Some may be warm and lively, their signals high; others cool and calm, their signals low. Ayurveda says this is no accident; these individual differences reflect each person's Prakriti, or body constitution, which is created and constantly influenced by the balance of the three doshas: Vata, Pitta, and Kapha.

Prakriti is the image that dies at the moment of conception, is implanted through the doshas of our parents, and is, in considerable measure, conditioned through the environment. It determines our appearance and how we think, feel, and experience health. Most Ayurvedic texts indicate that a deep understanding of Prakriti enables us to predict our natural propensities and weaknesses and make lifestyle choices that keep us in balance.

The five constituent elements of Prakriti are Vata, Pitta, and Kapha, which result from the five universal elements- air and space, fire and water, and earth and water, respectively. We predominate all three doshas in our system, though one or two predominantly rule, usually defining our body constitution. Among them are seven Prakriti types: single dosha dominating, i.e., Vataja, Pittaja, Kaphaja, dual dosha dominating or, Vata-Pitta, Pitta-Kapha, and Vata-Kapha, and a rare perfectly balanced type in which all the three Doshas are in equilibrium.

- **Dosha Imbalance: Causes and Symptoms**

Imagine being at the pinnacle of your health yet feeling something was a little out of kilter- a twinge of nausea, perhaps a touch of impending doom that eluded your nervous logical identification. In so many instances, this would suffice to act as the first stirrings that one of your doshas was out of balance. The balance of Vata, Pitta, or Kapha is disturbed by what one eats and what does not, the way of living and with whom, climate, and stress.

- **Vata Imbalance:** Vata is responsible for movement, manages the nervous system, and has the characteristics of lightness, dryness, and coldness. One shows symptoms of restlessness, anxiety, dry skin, constipation, and irregular appetite. For those with a predominant constitution of Vata, it would be easier to fall out of balance with too much exposure to cold, excessive travel, and eating erratically.

- **Pitta Imbalance:** Pitta is hot and sharp, associated with transformation and digestion. When Pitta goes off balance, one becomes overly critical, even angry, or has heartburn, rashes, or overheating. Since excessive Pitta has risen, this may ignite anger easily, especially in Pitta constitution types, because of feeling too hot, eating spicy food, or under undue tension.

- **Kapha Imbalance:** Kapha is heavy, calm, and stable. An imbalance may cause inertia, feelings of lethargy, accumulation of extra fat, congestion, and emotional resistance. Since kapha types are inactive, they are easily imbalanced by cold, damp weather, overeating, and lack of activity.

Relevant in this respect is to note that while our constitution or Prakriti does not alter during our lifetime, the three doshas - dependent on what surrounds us in life - are such: Vata, Pitta, and Kapha. Therefore, the knowledge of your Prakriti will amount to knowing when your doshas are out of step and what proper measures you must take to restore harmony.

- **Vata, Pitta, and Kapha: How to Know Your Body Type**

It is as if discovering a key was the principal way of knowing oneself better: by defining the body type or Prakriti. Each dosha is conceived to embody generic physical, emotional, and mental traits that reveal its elemental nature. Let's understand how to trace which dosha predominates in your constitution.

- **Vata Type: Air + Space**

People of the Vata type have lean, light bodies with a thin and tall physique. They have dry skin, coarse hair, and small, active eyes. They may never be able to gain weight quickly, eat less but frequently, have a low tolerance for cold weather, and tend to have cold hands and feet

- **Mental and Emotional Traits:** Vata is creative, curious, and quick to grasp and forget. This particular energy comes in spurts for this type—it is spontaneous, fast-paced, and talkative, and love and fear come quickly.

- **Imbalances:** When out of balance, the Vata types are insomnia-prone, anxious, and have dry skin, superficial veins, and indigestion. Their busy minds overwhelm them and make them feel scattered or restless.

- **Pitta Type: Fire + Water**

They have a medium build, warm, and shining skin. They sweat and urinate often, their skin and hair are oily, and their eyes are sharp. Early greying or baldness might be in the family, as might a sharp appetite and intolerance for hot weather. They may like to eat more frequently.

- **Mental and Emotional Traits:** Pittas are goal-oriented and sharp-witted, and we have a low tolerance for sharp-wittedness. They quickly become leaders and work well under pressure; thus, they tend toward goal-directed behavior. However, they can become irritable under stress and angry.
- **Imbalances:** Excessive Pitta can lead to inflammation, acidity, or skin rashes. Psychologically, people get overly critical or frustrated if they don't get what they want.

- **Kapha Type [Earth + Water] :**

The physiological characteristics of kapha types define them as well-built, with a wide and broad frame. Their muscles are also firm and well-developed. Their skin is usually soft, smooth, and cool to the touch. Their hair is thick and lustrous. They quickly gain weight, have strong joints, are tolerant of heat and hunger, and tend to have a slow metabolism.

- **Mental and Emotional Traits:** Kapha is calm, quiet, determined, patient, thinks before acts, and supportive.
- **Imbalances:** Any kapha imbalances causes weight gain, lethargy, congestion, and water retention. On the psyche's

level, it manifests as resistance or feeling stuck to new experiences.

So, you start understanding which dosha dominates in your constitution by observing physical traits, general tendencies of the mind, and how one responds in times of stress. Suppose you happen to be one of those who always feel cold, speak rapidly, and have dry skin; you fall into the category of Vata-dominant. And if you are always warm, sharp-brained, and quick to anger, then your principal dosha is probably Pitta. Your dominant dosha is probably Kapha if you are strong, sturdy, and slow to anger.

- **Conclusion: Soak Up Your Unique Constitution**

Therefore, the body's constitution is determined when the ovum meets the sperm, and its alignment and acceptance are the starting points toward living life in harmony and balance. "One size fits all" simply does not apply to health. Assessing the Ayurvedic body constitution type is crucial for determining appropriate treatment guidelines. For instance, if a person with a dominant pitta constitution is experiencing a Vata disorder, consuming hot properties in their diet and herbs could worsen the condition. Even though these hot properties may help pacify Vata, they could exacerbate pitta. Therefore, in such cases, it is advisable to use oils (sneha), heavy foods, and vata-pacifying herbs to subdue

You now know whether you are Vata, Pitta, or Kapha dominant and how that informs your understanding of how to live. A Prakriti examination should be followed by a Vikriti analysis to understand the nature and severity of illness, the prognosis of diseases, herbs that should be selected and administered, and diet and lifestyle changes to be recommended. The diet and lifestyle alteration recommendations should be based on diurnal and seasonal regimes.

You'll move through the world with energy, clarity, and calmness where your doshas are balanced.

Chapter 4: Mind—Mana, the Subtle Navigator

- **Concept of Mana or Mind and Its Importance in Ayurveda**

Standing at the shore of an endless ocean, a height-of-fascination moment, the breeze, the waves, and the horizon afar. Like the ocean, the mind is deep, comprehensive, and frequently cannot be calculated upon. According to Ayurveda, Mana or mind is a navigating vessel that sails us through those very waters of life, emotion, and experience. While it not only gives the power of thought, it is also the seat of perception whereby everything gets processed in this world, from outer stimuli to the innermost thoughts.

While the body one can easily see and touch, the mind cannot. Though the mind governs our actions and emotions, at times, we cannot understand the workings of the mind. In Ayurveda, any knowledge about the mind has to be understood, including the underlying forces at play within the subtle forces of our inner world and how they come into play with the outside world. According to the foremost scholar of Ayurveda, Sage Charak, the mind is mediated between Aatma and the senses. Only when the three come together can there be wisdom and understanding; when the mind strays, our vision regarding reality also becomes defective.

Let us illustrate how the mind works in daily life. You are in an office meeting in a restaurant. You hear the background noise of the cutlery and the chatter of people around you. But your mind only combines with your colleague's talk, so you hear only what your teammate says.

Even though you hear the background noise, you do not perceive it because your mind does not take that information. The mind develops knowledge or shuts it off according to the focus of concentration. The sages have illustrated the mind as minute/atomic and one rather than vast and many, which prevents the mind from obtaining a variety of knowledge at the moment.

It is so that the mind integrates sensory information and works on its meaning to enable us to make decisions and act upon them. However, all this does not happen by its own accord. Thus, if one is disturbed emotionally or the mind is not focused, the mind can play tricks. But when it's out of balance, we reach for harmful foods, strike out at others, or indulge in behaviors we know don't serve us well. That's why balancing the mind is Ayurveda's number one principle- not just to, affect our mental clarity but also to affect our physical and emotional health.

- **Balancing the Mind for Healthy Prospersance**

Mental health and medical diseases are also concerns for Ayurveda. A healthy mind forms the basis of good health. A balanced mind always produces a peaceful and serene feeling. Once the mind is perturbed, it destroys thoughtfulness and one's health.

Living in today's world means that we are always hooked to some form of technology and information, which is much more challenging to deal with so far as maintaining mental balance is concerned. Social media affects us at a deep level of the psyche. Humans find themselves comparing against others, bringing about feelings of inadequacy, envy, or guilt. Otherwise, we have inhaled emotions, not even our own, while scrolling endlessly-just about like everyone else. And that is where Gyan comes in.

Gyan in Ayurveda means understanding yourself and realizing how a situation, people, or even social media is making you feel. It is awareness about how one reacts to situations and emotions. You must have felt irritated seeing your friend's pictures of his vacation when, in fact, everything else was just okay the whole day. That is the mind reacting to something on the outside of it. With Gyan, you learn to look at these reactions and not get overwhelmed. It's the first step toward mental balance.

But self-awareness is half the battle won. Ayurveda is prescribed for Dhairya, which is patience and perseverance. For most of us, we live in a world of instant gratification. Patience is a virtue in scarce supply. We want success in our career now. We want to improve our health now. We want happiness in our relationships now. But to slow down, have faith in the process, and not get ruffled if things don't happen as scheduled is equally essential. Trust the process; be patient. The goal could be achieved without those heartaches and cold sweats.

Generally speaking, people want to lose pounds. Ayurveda would substitute crash diets, excruciatingly hard workouts, and a mad scramble to show results as fast as possible. It urges patience and steady habits that respect the body's rhythms while knowing that real change takes time. That very much fully applies to mental health—to manage stress, overcome anxiety, or break any negative habits, patience toward long-term balance is required.

The other Ayurvedic principle to follow to find mental stability is Satvavajay Chikitsa-a, a type of therapy directed at pacifying the mind. This could be meditation, mindfulness, or simply spending time in nature. A restless mind craves excitement; it jumps from thought to thought. Satvavajay Chikitsa helps the mind quiet down and return to its stillness position. For instance, spending time with your hobbies, outdoor visitation, or a simple walk in the park on a routine day is appealing and soothing to the mind.

- **How to apply Yogic principles in mental health**

Theoretically, the Ayurvedic and yogic concepts of mental health hold samadhi, or deep absorption of meditation, as the ultimate state of yogic practice within a mindfulness practice framework. In essence, it has been a potent intervention in keeping with the flux of the mind at an everyday level.

Now, put in an executive who is supposed to answer emails, attend meetings, and work with a team. The mind now jumps all over this way and that, just to keep up with everything. In one instance, no human can pay attention to more than one thing. Multitasking is a mere myth. At any given time, the mind could dwell on only one thing.

That's like threading a needle into a bunch of lotus petals. The needle pierces multiple layers of petals but only goes through one at any moment. The process of obtaining knowledge is so fast that we do not realize the time difference. In the same way, when it comes to paying attention to more than one thing, the mind flips back and forth between these things rapidly. Therefore, the mind can't correctly understand any one thing's details. This sets off a vicious circle of mental fatigue, low productivity, and rising levels of stress.

As the concept of presence in Yogic philosophy explains, if one were to center his attention to the present for wholesome involvement-whatever that may be, be it work, conversation, or having a meal-if the mind was on the present, there would be better clarity and less psychological dust, which increases not only our efficiency but also our peace. You could see how minutes passed when you were engrossed in an activity. That is the magic of working mindfulness. This mindfulness practice can make you far more effective and bring loads of calmness into your life.

The second psychological health principle, according to Ayurveda and yoga, is that mind, ego (Ahankaar), and intelligence (Buddhi) have to work in harmony. The ego typically drags us towards appreciation, success, or pleasure, while intelligence helps explain what is in a person's best interest. The mind fluctuates between these two forces and chooses what the senses represent. For example, on the one hand, your senses want a dessert. On the other hand, the intellect says I must not have too much sugar. That is how a war is born inside the brain and helps you choose one alternative. The lamp's wick absorbs the oil and generates light, similar to how the senses take in information and pass it to the mind. The mind makes decisions and then passes them to the ego, which asserts its authority and passes the information to intelligence.

- **How to nourish your mind through Ayurvedic Routines**

Ayurveda has a lot of equipment and practices that are advised for the caretaking and balancing of the mind. Meditation is the most potent tool for soothing the mind and keeping any stress at a distance. If meditation is done by either breathing or with a mantra, it quietens the eternal chattering that is going on within the mind and brings it to a state of stillness. Regular meditation Gradually makes one much more resilient against stress and other emotional challenges.

Pranayama, or breathing exercises, help the mind keep its balance. The interrelationship between the breath and mind is such that the mind flickers when one breathes fast and shallowly. In contrast, if one breathes slowly and more profoundly, it automatically calms down. Practices like Anulom Vilom (Alternate nostril breathing) or Bhramari (humming bee breath) soothe the nervous system and help lessen anxiety.

Some extracts are known to have a calming effect on the nervous system, thus keeping the mind in excellent health. Shankhpushpi is one of the best examples; this, an Ayurvedic herb, has been used for several years for cooling the brain and improving concentration. It forms part of treatments that are instrumental in treating patients prone to anxiety, depression, and insomnia. Shankapushpi, taken with milk and added with a pinch of turmeric, acts like a very potent tonic (rasayana) for the mind and keeps the mind sharp and clear.

- **Conclusion: The Attainment of a Quiet and Concentrated Mind**

The mind is strong, fragile, and able to create incredible creativity, solve dilemmas, determine the probability of something being successful, and recognize emotions and insight. It can easily be set aflutter by emotional turbulence. According to Ayurveda, this subtle captain navigates life through all the various complexities in the world. A balanced mind implies clarity, focus, and calm of all things. Disturb it, and everything suffers- physical health, emotions, and relationships.

The more we learn to cultivate awareness, patience, and mindfulness, the more quickly we will surmount all the difficulties in life. Just as the body requires food and rest, the mind also requires other kinds of practice, such as meditation, breathing, and introspection, to keep balance.

Further in the journey of Ayurveda, remember that caretaking of the mind works precisely as one does for one's body. Thus, when provided with the right tools and practices, he or she can keep his mind composed, sharp, and resilient towards all odds.

Chapter 5: Soul—Aatma: The Eternal Witness

The Soul Cycle: Ayurveda

There is silence within us, silently watching all the turmoil of life go by. Is the Aatma the soul that cannot be shaken, never-changing, untouchable by time or circumstance, but in constant motion? With every change in body, in mind, with every tide of fortune and ill, the soul stands unmoved, alert, and watchful. It cannot fade, grow weary, or sag. It is that which has been always, is now, and ever shall be.

"Ayurveda teaches that 'the soul is the keystone around which all of life pivots.'". Conceptions in the West view the body as the ultimate purpose of life. In contrast, Ayurveda looks at the body merely as a temporary abode for the soul-it houses her for one lifetime only before moving on. The soul remains indelibly marked with impressions from past lives, and it crosses over, one body to another, exploring the world in all the shapes and sizes it takes on. While these bodies come and go and die, the soul endures, freed by the cleansing of the influence of the material world. This soul journey in a birth, death, and rebirth cycle is called Samsara.

Think about this: the body you walk in today is not one your soul has lived in before and certainly will not be the last. Each life is a new lesson, experience, and chance to learn. The soul is always learning for balance, understanding, and liberation. In Ayurveda, the term is known as Moksha, which means freedom from the cycle of Samsara and emergence into universal consciousness, free from worldly entanglements and desires.

Relationship between Soul, Mind and Sense

A delicate dance between the soul, the mind, and the senses defines our human experience. The soul is the silent witness, the mind interprets, and the senses relate to the world. The union of the senses with the soul gives us the fabric of our reality.

Recall times when you felt connected to the moment: perhaps by the awe of being before sunset or the quiet delight of being embraced by a loved one. Here, the soul bonds with the world through the senses, but the mind bridges the senses and the soul. The senses steal in what we perceive, hear, taste, and touch; the mind can interpret it, and the soul silently absorbs what is sharply cutting each moment.

This, though, is a fragile bond. Knowledge is not perceived by being mind-distracted, filled with negative thoughts, or when the feelings are not pure. Just as a person can't see their face in the muddy waters of a lake, the mess of the mind muddles the soul's contact with the world. Says Ayurveda, it is this 'new-mind freshness,' freed from negativity, that will permit the soul to connect thoroughly with the senses and experience which we can get peace, joy, or awareness.

In this respect, the mind, intellect (Buddhi), and senses are the instruments that merge with the soul to allow actions to happen. One of the mind's significant responsibilities is steering the senses toward balance. Without it, the senses will lead us astray into excesses of pleasure or away from needed challenges. When the mind is free of distortion, it can open itself to allow the soul to understand life as it is given its fullness.

The Eternal vs. the Impermanent

We indeed live in a world where, by nature, everything seems to be impermanent: the body grows old; friendship becomes what perhaps it never was; a career is winding down, and even the closest relationships blow with the wind. So easily bogged down by the impermanence, by the fixation on what we shall lose and what's going to shift next, Ayurveda says it is all about looking beyond that transience to see what is permanent.

The soul is eternal and known as Anadi purusha. It lacks a beginning and can not be logically understood. The soul is constant, permanent, expressionless, without reasons, and not associated with hate or desire. This eternalness can not be expressed, perceived, or thought about.

The soul is all-pervading, perpetual, and forever. It can never be destroyed, cannot be perceived by the senses, and, therefore, cannot be expressed. The sages have said that actions in this world have a reason, and just as we imagine a creator for the world whom we do not see, a soul is an imagination that exists.

The Being as Impermanent: The creation of a being (purusha) is based on certain causes-attachment, desire, likes/dislikes. The one created with reasons, such as the being (purusha), is impermanent. The body is impermanent; it is born, grows, decays, and dies. That is, the character of the mind also changes its emotions, thoughts, and the impressions it bears. Yet the soul changes not at all. This is an immortal constituent of our life experience that nothing in this world or this life has ever touched. The earthly body aches grows old, and dies. The soul suffers not on these grounds. It watches; it is indifferent to the dramatics of life.

This consciousness changes our way of living, seeing that if we realize that the body and mind are impermanent, we should let go of the transients of life we live. We begin to accept whatever change comes our way because we understand that only the soul matters. The things that too often fill our heads with fear and anxiety-aging, loss, and failure, will now lose their hold on us once we have realized that. Indeed, these are but momentary.

There is great peace in this. Think of the experience with life's problems, disappointment, uncertainty-and knowing this will be but waves on an ocean that will pass. And it keeps quiet, like deep water below the surface and with all the turmoil as that may be above in the waves. That's the eternally spiritual nature of the soul, and it is one of the most precious gifts Ayurveda gives to us- that no matter what may happen in life, we remain the same as our soul and, hence, cannot change.

This also makes life easier and more gracious. In one way, it allows one to experience the transition from fear and attachment to peace and acceptance. Thus, one learns to let go of the temporal and embrace the eternal, moving toward the final freedom and truth of the soul.

Conclusion: Life in the Presence of the Soul

It is because it is our eternal witness, within us, unchanged in the maelstrom and turmoil of life. And it is only through knowing the journey of the soul, its relation to mind and senses, that we may live with more peace, knowing what never will and must pass. Ayurvedic soul teachings are not about extrication from life but how to live more meaningfully. The knowledge that one's soul lives eternally keeps a person more present, compassionate, and receptive to the deeper rhythms of life. We learn that such difference is not between lightning flash and perpetual light, but between life and death, between the fleeting and the eternal, between the mistake of the transitory and the infinite flight of the soul-a flight that transcends at once both body and mind, stretching beyond time toward a last end: liberation.

Remember, a soul is always there for you, silently seeing and guiding, waiting for you to acknowledge them. And that acknowledgment is the answer to a peaceful, purposeful, and fulfilling life.

Chapter 6: The Seven Pillars - Dhatus of Life

A human is not just the form of a physical, biological entity but an inner, conscious being. In this vast ocean of Ayurvedic knowledge, the dhatus represent the foundation upon which our body is erected, maintained, and sustained. As we know, the word "dhatu" literally means "that which supports" or "upholder." That is precisely what the seven dhatus do - they are the upholders of the human body; they bring nourishment and sustenance to it. They are behind our growth, strength, and even vitality. Furthermore, they form the very base of a healthy body. To understand what dhatus are is to know intricately how our body functions and thrives.

Seven dhatus form what in Ayurveda is known as the Annamaya Kosha, or physical sheath of the body, being the most material layer of our existence. They undertake various jobs but collectively keep the human body balanced and healthy. Food nourishes them; if well cared for, they give us strength, power, and general well-being. However, when it degenerates or is otherwise disordered-most often through poor diet or other inappropriate lifestyles, the entire system can be thrown into chaos.

The Seven Dhatus: An Overview

The Ayurvedic model emphasizes the seven dhatus or tissues constituting the body's integrity and health. Seven dhatus include Rasa (plasma), Rakta (blood), Mamsa (muscle), Meda (fat), Asthi (bone), Majja (bone marrow), and Shukra (reproductive tissue) -each having independent functions.

They are interdependent; one feeds the other in an exact and sequential order. This process is termed Dhatu Parinama, whereby the nutrients from digested food become nutrition and support for each dhatu.

Plasma is the direct outcome of digestion. Thus, it imparts moisture to all the other dhatus and is full of energy and power.

- Rasa dhatu: It gives the body and skin a glow and balances emotions. It helps the body stay grounded and brings satisfaction to the mind (mana).
- Rakta Dhatu or Blood: It performs oxygenation to the body; thus, a nourishing agent is delivered to muscle and skin elements. Therefore, the complexion is strongly supported by rakta dhatu. Healthy rakta dhatu will give you a rosy glow and make you intelligent, energetic, and eager to take action.
- Mansa Dhatu (Muscle Tissue): It delivers strength and body structure. It lubricates the body and makes up the most significant portion of our gross physical body. It produces sweat and strengthens the bones and the body.
- Meda dhatu (fat tissue): It is an internal layer that lubricates the skin, joints, and organs. It covers the body internally, keeping it warm and serving as a reserve for energy. In return, the proper balance of meda dhatu balances body weight and softens the body by lubricating and producing sweat.
- Asthi Dhatu (Bone tissue): It forms the body's framework, supporting and stabilizing it. Good, healthy, and strong asthi dhatu provides good, strong bones, teeth, and nails.
- Majja Dhatu (Bone Marrow and Nerve Tissue): It fills the bones and fuels the nervous system. It also constitutes cognitive functions and sharp thought. Healthy Majja dhatu

gives strength and passion for love and nourishes the reproductive tissue.

- Shukra Dharu (reproductive tissue): The last dhatu is the most subtle, the Shukra dhatu, involved in sexual desires and procreation. It is the essence of vivacity and creativity. Well-nourished Shukra dhatu supports and enhances healthy reproductive functions, vitality, and virility.

Functions and Nutrition of Each Dhatu

Each dhatu plays a specific role that is more than simple physical functions. All these functions interconnect with the healthiness of our minds and emotions. This is how each of these dhatus can be nourished through dietary and lifestyle modification:

Rasa Dhatu

Function: Nourishment, hydration, and energy

Nutrition: Hydration foods, those which contain large amounts of water, like fresh fruits, soups, and juices, nourish the Rasa dhatu. Proper hydration that moistens the body is the means of maintaining Rasa in equilibrium.

Rakta Dhatu

Function: It oxygenates the body and energizes and colors the tissues. It is also associated with the passion and energy of activity.

Nutrition: Iron-rich foods like green leafy vegetables, beetroot, pomegranates, and lentils suit Rakta dhatu. Turmeric, cumin, and other spices help cleanse blood and improve circulation.

Mamsa Dhatu

Function: It builds up muscles and provides strength and architecture to the body.

Nutrition: Protein-rich foods like lentils, beans, nuts, and whole grains are good for Mamsa Dhatu, and strength training supports it.

Meda Dhatu

Function: It protects the physical body and contains immediate sources of energy.

Nutrition: An adequate balance in Meda Dhatu is always achieved by eating healthy fats like ghee, avocado, chia seeds, flax seeds, olive oil, and avocado oil. The accumulation of excess fat can always be managed by taking moderate amounts of food.

Asthi Dhatu

Function: It provides structure to and supports the body's skeletal system, strengthening the bones and teeth.

Nutrition: Calcium-dairy foods, including sesame seeds, leafy greens, and almonds. Exposure to the sun for at least 15 minutes provides vitamin D for strong bones.

Majja Dhatu

Function: It strengthens the bone marrow and nervous system and enhances cognitive functions and emotional equilibrium.

Nutrition: Flaxseeds, chia seeds, walnuts, and fish rich in omega-3. These nourish the brain and the nervous system. Meditative practices and soothing habits nurture Majja dhatu by bringing serenity to the mind and emotions.

Shukra Dhatu

Function: Supports Sexual Wellbeing, Energy, and Creativity

Nutrition: Shukra Dhatu's nutrition includes dairy, almonds, dates, and asparagus racemosus (shatavari). Healthy sleep, balanced physical exercise, and an affectionate and nourishing environment promote its production.

Maintenance Diet for the Dhatus

Dhatus should be adequately maintained and harmoniously. Agni- the digestive fire- digests food and converts it into necessary nutrient sources that contribute to the sustenance of each dhatu. Any diet would suffice, provided it is suited to one's prakriti and current state of health. The characteristics of the recommended foods are fresh, seasonal, and easy to digest. Cooking with digestive spices such as cumin, coriander, and ginger further increases Agni and facilitates proper digestion.

General guidelines for maintaining the health of the dhatus

A diet that contains all six tastes: sweet, sour, salty, bitter, spicy, and astringent provides a variety of nutrients for each of the dhatu to function properly and harmoniously.

Drink ample water, but ensure it is warm or at room temperature. Cold water can depress Agni. It is advised that one stops eating when they are satiated.

Conclusion: Dhatus as the base of Health

Dhatus are the pillar upon which our health stands. The dhatu's nutrition is a prime requirement for maintaining balance in our system. This way, by knowing how to work each of the dhatus and what it requires to maintain their health, we could take an active role towards our health so that we do not just survive but, more than that, truly live and thrive. Such a person, kept in shape and harmony by mindful eating and balanced and conscious living, with awareness over their body needs, can support the dhatus and thereby be able to enjoy life vibrant and in balance.

Chapter 7: Ojas – The Vital Fluid Component

What is Ojas?

There is that person who walks into the room, and you feel their energy and presence. Yet they haven't said a word. They radiate an aura of power and calm. It's that unspoken, undefined quality, this glow. It's more than health; it is the life force, the vital energy. This is called Ojas in Ayurveda.

In Ayurveda, Ojas is described as the subtle essence that ties together physical, mental, and spiritual wellness. Often, it has been described as the "vital fluid component" or the "essence of all the dhatus," which was dealt with in-depth in the previous chapter. Ojas are said to be produced when the body's tissues are well-nourished and balanced, making for radiant health. It can be compared with the nectar of life, which is the final product of well-digested food, a well-balanced mind, and a peaceful spirit. When we have a lot of Ojas, we are alive, energetic, and strong, and we can conveniently face the challenges in life.

However, Ojas is fragile. Any kind of stress, bad food, negative thoughts, or overexertion could cause it to wind down, leaving us depleted, nervous, too dry, and open to illness. Candlelight protects and keeps it alive, and it shines bright and radiantly. But as stronger forces attack it, it keeps flickering and smothering with the slightest draft.

Immunity and Vitality: The role of Ojas

Ojas has to do with immunity and vitality. Sages conceptualized the residence of Ojas in the heart, where the seat of one type of Pitta-

Sadhak Pitta- is also present. The sages also indicate that the Ojas are the ultimate pure vital component that can not be seen, similar to the concept of a soul. Ojas supports the body with lubrication and purity. When our Ojas are fine, our defense mechanisms are in the pink of health, we have a great complexion, diseases are at bay, and we recover from illness. But it's not just physical strength; Ojas also rules mental and emotional stamina. It gives us the resilience and courage to deal with difficult times, the patience to cope with stress, and the emotional equilibrium to maintain healthy relationships.

Imagine the concept of Ojas as fuel for the body's immune system. If the body is nourished and the lifestyle is well-balanced, the body naturally has ample fuel for peak immune system performance. Once that Ojas runs out, it's like running an immune system without fuel, making one more prone to infections, fatigue, and chronic diseases.

Consider Meera. On paper, she is everything a woman could ever want: a career catapulting her success, a wonderful family, and an active social life. Over time, as she does more and more at work, she eats less often, sleeps less usually, and increasingly takes off the edge. She tends to remain angry and irritable at her kids and overthinks about unnecessary issues. At first, everything went well, but soon, something was wrong. She would catch a cold easily for months, always remained tired, and her head foggy. Still, despite all her achievements, she feels completely drained and can’t work as hard anymore. Meera's story is an episode of Ojas's exhaustion. Her body overexertion and a lack of self-caring have left her vulnerable as her reservoirs of Ojas have been spent.

Ojas protects us against physical illness and nurture our emotional and mental energy. When the levels are high, it makes us solid, composed, clear-headed, and joyful. It supports our muscles, cartilage, and bones and strengthens our body. Then, we can face all life's adversities with equanimity, motivation, and gratitude and not get drowned in the storms of life. When it falls off, we are anxious, fearful, tense for no reason, and sad most of the time. Not that it's a question of fighting off colds but of keeping the inner strength to thrive despite stress.

Building Up Ojas through Lifestyle and Diet

Fortunately, conscious lifestyle and diet choices can strengthen and enhance Ojas. Ayurveda offers a wealth of tools to protect and reinforce Ojas so we are healthy and deeply nourished. Let's explore how this life force could be enhanced daily.

- 1. Foods that Nourish Ojas

Our diet directly impacts the quality of our Ojas. Pure, fresh, and light foods feed them; processed, heavy, or artificial foods weaken them. A Sattvic diet that is pure, light, and energizing builds strong Ojas: fresh fruits and vegetables, whole grains, nuts and seeds, dairy, and naturally sweet items like dates and honey.

For instance, ghee is one of the most decadent foods for building Ojas. It is so nourishing that it digests quickly, lubricates, and strengthens all body tissues. Almonds and walnuts soaked overnight and peeled are also excellent food for Ojas. They have an extremely high nutrient value and support physical and mental energy.

An age-old remedy for building Ojas is a warm glass of milk with a pinch of cardamom, turmeric, or saffron. The body becomes strong, but the mind becomes soft.

The key point to remember here is how to eat: how matters as much as what. We should take and savor every bite mindfully, in calm surroundings, and treat the body appropriately to digest and assimilate those nutrients. Such eating will help us derive as much nourishment as possible, which will feed our Ojas immediately.

- 2. Rest

Stress and overwork are among the quickest drains on the Ojas. In a society that prides itself on being "busy," it becomes easy to forget how vital rest is to building and protecting the Ojas.

One of the finest ways to replenish Ojas is through adequate, rejuvenating sleep. This is the time for our body and mind to mend, revive, and gather new energy for the new day's activities ahead. Ayurveda recommends sleeping for 7 to 8 hours undisturbed at night. One should ideally go to bed early and wake up with the sun. Any sleep ritual should be devoid of screen usage, with relaxing activities like light stretches, a warm bath, or a cup of herbal tea that might help one sleep deeply and soundly.

But rest is not merely sleep. It's also the space of the mind. Meditation, yoga, and simple breathing exercises soothe the mind, reduce stress, and bring inner peace that brings about Ojas. Indeed, time spent in nature, far away from the heavy weight of modern life, also rejuvenates Ojas. Whether it is a walk in the park, sitting by the ocean, or merely viewing the garden's beauty, nature brings about a sense of serenity and revivifies the vital energies of our being.

- 3. Positive Feelings and Clarity of Mind

Just as negative emotions such as anger, fear, and anxiety deplete Ojas, positive emotions build it back up. A feeling of gratefulness, compassion, and joy can nourish a sense of emotional wellness and fortify the composition of Ojas directly. One's surroundings and the people they have in their environment can make a lot of difference in the longevity of mental and emotional vitality. Being surrounded by inspirational people with whom you're ready to share meaningful conversations and find time to enjoy hobbies and various creative outlets can make a lot of therapeutic difference.

Mindfulness of what we do to and with our daily fare while eating, working, and socializing keeps us connected to the present. Being immersed in the moment, without looking ahead or worrying about what's following, naturally protects and builds up Ojas. This lends itself to an easy passage in life with ample ease and grace and sometimes stops mental and emotional friction that can cause energy loss.

- 4. Balancing Activity and Rest

While physical exertion is an integral part of a healthy life, overexertion can lead to the waste of Ojas. Ayurvedic physicians also prescribe equilibrium between exercising and resting. Balanced living—walking, yoga, or swimming—improves energy flow and helps the body without stress. In contrast, overworking the body is said to consume Ojas if it is not coupled with proper rest and nutrition.

Ayurveda teaches us to respect our natural rhythms. This can be reflected in nature's cycles of days and nights, seasons and growth, and there are cycles in our bodies as well. If we listen to those, our balance will be strong enough to build Ojas. This may be difficult work when needed, but we should slow down and recharge ourselves when we feel our energy depleted.

Conclusion: Living with Ojas

Ojas is not only a word in Ayurveda. Once again, our inner essence, invisible energy, makes us healthy, joyful, and resilient. Good care for our Ojas makes us feel more vital, earthed, and connected with ourselves and the world around us.

Building Ojas is not easy; it takes time to build up. This can only be done by conscious choice-making in diet, rest, relationships, and care for body and mind. What are the rewards? When we have good Ojas, everything falls into place; the day-to-day challenges of life are faced more easily, health is preserved, and there is a more profound feeling of peace and well-being.

The world invites us to be more, do more, and go faster, but Ayurveda extends precisely this invitation—an invitation to stop, listen to the body, and water the quiet power of Ojas. In slowing down, in being mindful of it, lies the true essence of vitality.

Chapter 8: Yukti - The Art and Science of Healing

- **Understanding Yukti in Ayurvedic Practice**

Ayurveda healing is not simply doling out herbs or checking off lists. It is an art—a subtle balance of science and intuition whereby the practitioner harmonizes her intellect with her wisdom. This skill is called Mukti. With this skill, treatments may be applied thoughtfully and creatively according to the peculiar needs of the patient.

Imagine a musician playing a song. Whereas with music in front of them, it is, in fact, all about the play- the emotion they bring, how they feel the movement or the flow of the melody- that mastery is seen. Similarly, an Ayurvedic healer would use their wisdom to change treatments based on the constitution of the patient's strength, the season, the environment, and the individual's emotional state. Yukti is the intuition of the healer- the ability developed over the years that lets him see beyond the visible symptoms and treat the primary causes of sickness.

Yukti cannot be attained by reading books. It's born from practice, observation, and a deep understanding of the human body. Ancient sages understood this; they knew that knowing about herbs or treatments was not enough. It is about knowing when and how to apply this knowledge, adapting to the situation, and healing.

- **Application of Ayurveda in Treatment**

Ayurveda treatments are highly individualistic. Two patients suffering from the same ailment will be treated entirely and diametrically differently depending on their constitution or Prakriti. For example, an aggravation of Vata could well cause one person's anxiety, while an excess of Pitta could cause it in another. Therefore, Yukti will ensure that the healer understands and treats these differences accordingly.

Let's take an example of a patient with joint pains. A book text advises certain herbs, but the practitioner knows that in cold, damp winters, that particular herb is of little use to a Kapha-dominating individual. Instead, they would choose a warming herb to fight off the cold aggravating the joints. Yukti in action: one deals with the individual and disease, not just the disease.

It becomes apparent in the following situation: sometimes, Yukti comes into play when there isn't enough. The herb one wants to use isn't in season or geographically abundant. A wise practitioner knows to substitute another herb that shares the qualities available so the treatment will still be effective. That ability to pivot and shift thinking is the difference between a good healer and an excellent one. This adaptability and knowledge let Ayurveda flow smoothly across cultures, climates, and times.

- **Case studies in healing with Yukti**

Let's take Joe, a middle-aged male patient who spent his days all down with chronic fatigue. He underwent almost every alternative medicine and lifestyle change he could think of, but still, he felt that this thing was not going very well. It was when he finally consulted an

Ayurvedic practitioner, who was not only bothered about his ailment but went ahead to analyze his daily regime, mental state, and food intake. Joe's state of affairs was more complex than simply digestive problems but, instead, emotional stress over years that hadn't been dealt with.

The practitioner did combinations of treatments through soothing herbs for his digestive system, meditation practice targeting the cause of stress, and a nourishing diet to build up the remaining energy reserve. Slowly but surely, vitality returned to Joe. It wasn't just the herbs-it was seeing the whole picture and applying treatments that reached his mind, body, and soul.

Another example is of a woman, Meena, who, when seen by an Ayurvedic doctor, presented with very severe skin rashes. The doctor inquired about her constitution and diagnosed that time was at the peak of summer. Thus, the doctor found the Pitta of Meena very highly aggravated. She is considered an exception rather than a standard case; the healer changed her treatment to add pitta, balancing herbs and activities such as not consuming spicy foods and staying in the sun to regain her inner balance because she was overheated. Gradually, she recovered, and the skin healed with time.

- **Conclusion: The Mastery of Yukti**

Yukti is what differentiates a good healer from a great one. The ability, for example, not just to see the person but also to take on the moment and to make sense by intuitive choices that transcend the botanical knowledge, such as in the wisdom that sometimes healing has nothing to do with the herb but when, how, and what amount it is given. Ayurveda postulates that the healer's role is not limited to a prescription of treatment but the art, an intricate weaving of science, intuition, and experience, to figure out true healing when things are tough.

A good healer heals not only the illness but the person, and it's in that subtle, delicate balance that the actual depth of Yukti lies.

SECTION-2

Chapter 9: Embracing Daytime Rhythms—Dincharya and Ratricharya

We live today in such a hectic world that we tend to go about our day without any real awareness of natural rhythms guiding us: We eat when it is convenient, sleep when we feel exhausted, and very rarely pay attention to what our daily routines might be causing in terms of health. This section of Ayurveda defines what daily rituals are called Dincharya and Ratricharya, and it is posited that these are seminal sectors of being in balance and, therefore, health in the body and the mind. So, if we apply activity to our natural hours of daylight and darkness, we can expand our body health and the clarity of our emotional and mental selves.

- **Daily Ritual for Sound Health and Harmony**

Let's begin with the morning when the key to a healthy day starts as early as sunrise. According to Ayurveda, it is worthwhile to get up before dawn. What is projected into this rising should match the rising Vata energy that occurs precisely early, with all its lightness and clarity. This is an excellent opportunity to set the direction of your day.

We need to drink water as soon as we wake up. Hydration has much to do with it, but that's not all; these are jump-starting body systems, digestions moving gently and smoothly, and, most importantly, the doshas regulating drinking water. Drinking 16 oz of water at around 5:30 or 6:00 am will do good to the body, not aging too young, proper health within digestion, and even letting piles, digestive disorders, and edema calm down. This is a straightforward yet effective practice to clean the body inside.

Perhaps the most frequently abused is evacuation. Urine and bowel movements in the morning ought to flush out toxins in the body and help jumpstart the day. Even if you do not feel like it, this habit trains the body to make this a conditioned response during the morning.

- **Natural Rhythms: Living by Nature's Rules**

Ayurveda recommends some practices during the morning if you want your body to maintain balance. Oil pulling, also called Gandoosh, involves swishing oil in the mouth for some time. It strengthens the teeth and removes toxins from the body, hence good oral health and vitality in general.

The next important one is physical activity, which keeps the body and mind light and energized. Exercise stimulates digestive fire, increases appetite, reduces stress, keeps the muscles fit, and controls the amount of healthy fats. However, Ayurveda says exercise should not be overdone; otherwise, it will exhaust the reserve stored in the body. Gentle, regular movement keeps everything properly balanced.

An oil rub after exercise nourishes the body and the mind; it does. Massaging the body with warm oil increases circulation and relaxation, improving skin health. It is a very special ritual that works on the physical and emotional planes to connect the person with his body and offer a moment of mindfulness.

Following Abhyanga, the bath cleanses the body and revitalizes the mind. According to Ayurveda, heat balance is maintained in the body if warmer water is used below the waistline and cooler water is applied to the head. This refreshing bath strengthens the reproductive system, boosts enthusiasm, and cleanses the body of sweat and fatigue.

- **Day and Night Essentials for Health and Well-being**

Ayurveda prescribes gradually increasing the care with food during the day. This should provide its biggest meal in the middle of the day, coinciding with Pitta energy that peaks when the sun is high and is a precursor of potent digestive power. It would be the perfect time to have more substantial or more heavily prepared meals because the body's digestive power should be the highest during this period.

But the importance of Dincharya is not determined by the day. Evening brings Ratricharya, or nightly routines, are equally important for maintaining health.

A part of Ratricharya is that dinner should be eaten early—not later in the evening, as in many post-industrialized lifestyles. The dinner should be light and easily digestible; it should not be too heavy with oils, which may choke the digestive system and adversely affect sleep. After dinner, a slow walk of 100 steps is good practice. This helps the body digest food and calms it before sleep.

Ayurveda also recognizes the distinct healing qualities of nocturnal activities. A walk in the evening under a moonlit sky, mainly when the full moon is up, is said to pacify Pitta dosha. The lunar temperature cools any fire in the system and alleviates restlessness, thirst, and feverishness. It is said to soothe the mind, similar to when one feels satisfied after an intimate moment, as it gives a feeling of deep satisfaction and brings about tranquility.

Going to bed early is crucial for maintaining health and happiness. The attractiveness of staying up late may be offset by losing Kapha energy and increasing dryness in the body. The body tissues, or the dhatus, restore their balance during sleep, preparing the strength, stamina, and enthusiasm for the next day. If you sleep early, between 9:30 and 10:00 p.m., you can repair and rejuvenate.

Therefore, the third and final aspect of Ayurveda is listening to your body's natural urges. Whether it is the urge to let bowel pass, urinate, or sneeze, suppressing these urges creates imbalances and leads to illness. For instance, this would mean dizziness or perhaps heart problems while ignoring thirst and headaches while preventing sneezing. Observing your body signals immediately keeps you in tune with nature's rhythm and prevents discomfort later.

- **Conclusion: To Live in Accord with Nature**

Learn to live with nature by observing Dincharya and Ratricharya. Observe the laws of day and night. Such practices seem so simple yet fiercely shape health and energy. The secret is continuity of habits; the more one performs daily practice, the more it will help one gain better insight into the self and the world.

Life is not just about having a healthy body but also about living in balance, clarity, and deep peace. So, for example, let's have water immediately after we wake up, start having dinner early, retire to bed as early as possible, and do more such little and meaningful practices to upgrade our health and bring calmness into our daily lives.

These tested routines will improve energy, strengthen the digestive system, and orient the mind to peace. It's simply embracing life rhythms, allowing them to bring you more excellent health and happiness.

Chapter 10: Dancing with the Seasons—Ritucharya

There is a rhythm to life that goes beyond the sun's rising and setting and the ways of the turning seasons. In Ayurveda, this dance or rhythm is known as Ritucharya, the practice of aligning one's lifestyle, diet, and habits with the cycles of nature. Just like the earth, we change with each passing season. Learning to dance with changing times keeps us well grounded and disallows the sickness of imbalance.

- **Seasonal Changes and Health Effects**

According to Ayurveda, there are six seasons: Shishir, which refers to the late winter season; Vasant, the spring season; Grishma, summer; Varsha, the monsoon season; Sharad, the autumn season; and Hemant, the early winter season. All these seasons, with their unique climatic characteristics, impact not only the exterior environment but also strike within our very system regarding how things go regarding the three doshas: Vata, Pitta, and Kapha.

For example, on Shishir, a sign of the end of winter, the air is cold and dry; hence, it usually tends to produce an excess of Vata. The Agni, or digestive fire, becomes more potent in response to the cold; thus, we get hungry more during winter. Then, as far as the Vasant, or spring season, is concerned, it is said to produce Kapha in surplus quantities because of its moisture and lubricating qualities, causing people to be stagnant or congested at times.

And then there's Summer, or Grishma - a season of high heat that essentially increases Pitta. We get dehydrated and have skin problems, irritation, and headaches. Then, Varsha, or monsoon, brings in lots of coolness. That time, our tendency will increase Vata; honestly, we cannot resist weakening the digestion system; thus, it makes us helpless against problems like bloating and gas. The arrival of Sharad brings it only to the level of irritation in Pitta; however, Hemant-cooling things out like Shishir brings in the great desire for more nourishing food.

The simple principle of staying healthy throughout the year is to learn how each season affects the doshas. Anyone living and eating the same way every month of the year is out of step with nature's rhythms, and imbalances begin to manifest as health problems.

- **Seasonal Diet and Lifestyle Changes**

Ayurveda advises changing diet and lifestyle according to the season, just as clothes change according to the season. Let's learn how to change habits to keep well-balanced and fit throughout the year.

Shishir and Hemant (Late Winter and Early Winter)

The body craves something warm and nourishing when the sun stays north during winter. Cold raises Vata and feeds digestion. Winter can be an excellent time to indulge in heart-warming meals and culinary treats. Rich, nourishing foods that are just a little bit oily, like soups and stews, ghee, and warm oats, help counter the cold and dryness of winter.

Massages, such as Abhyanga with sesame oil, can be taken as a warm shower in the morning, keeping the body lubricated from the dryness of this season. Routine light exercise will keep Kapha from imbalance and prevent any slowness of movement from the cold.

- **Vasant (Spring)**

All that congestion, sluggish digestion, and even seasonal allergies are symptoms of increased Kapha within the body when the snow melts and the earth begins to wet. Lighter, cleansing foods, so Ayurveda teaches, are necessary to prepare for spring's heavy, sticky qualities: bitter greens, barley, honey, and Haritaki powder mixed with honey.

Detox practices like Vaman, or therapeutic vomiting to clear sinuses and the upper respiratory tract, and Nasya, or nasal oiling, are also in their perfect season. Spring is the time to get moving. Exercise becomes essential to prevent Kapha's buildup, so outdoor activities and morning walks are highly encouraged.

- **Grishma (Summer)**

Summer is hot—it's the season of Pitta intensity. Excessive heat can cause dehydration, irritation, and other problems. Cooling and hydrating foods are best for this. Cucumbers, watermelon, coconut water, kokum juice, lemon water, and leafy green vegetables can be your allies, cooling the body from within and helping you find an exact balance between the fire nature of Pitta.

Also, avoid heavy, spicy, oily foods because they irritate the Pitta dosha. Eat light food in your stomach and drink lots of water. Add cooling herbs like mint and coriander to buttermilk to pacify the heat.

Try to avoid exposure to bright sun rays during peak sun hours. Keep yourselves under shades and take cool showers. Spend some time resting in summer because that causes the body to fatigue most easily.

- **Varsha (Monsoon)**

The rainy season usually causes an imbalance of Vata because the atmosphere is calm, wet, and damp. Therefore, digestion weakens, making the body more productive but prone to burps and swelling. Ayurveda recommends warm, moist food that is easy to digest, like soups, stews, and porridges.

Raw, cold foods are no longer favored as they introduce plenty of Vata. To digest food well, spice it up with ginger, cumin, turmeric, etc., and include various tastes to brighten the digestive fire. Steam baths and saunas can facilitate flushing excess moisture out of the body.

- **Sharad (Autumn)**

Since Pitta is still active at the beginning of the second half of summer and slips into autumn, the Sharad season tries to cool down and soothe it through diet, which includes dairy, ghee, and cooling grains such as basmati rice. Overly spicy, salty, and sour foods will inflame Pitta further.

This will quiet down the standard emotional heat and irritation during this season.

- **Benefits of Prevention against Seasonal Diseases**

Other benefits of Ritucharya include prevention against seasonal diseases. Observing the Ayurveda seasonal guidelines enhances our body's natural defensive powers and prevents doshas from being aggravated.

For example, we drink plenty of fluids and eat delicious food in summer to avoid dehydration and heat stroke. Similarly, with the arrival of spring, following a detoxifying practice and consuming less food will serve the body as an oasis that escapes excess congestion and the slowness of Kapha.

As we swim along nature's rhythms, we make these seasonal adjustments to fine-tune our health and avoid the common ails that arise when we are out of sync with our environment. Seasonally appropriate foods, changes in physical activities according to seasons, and Ayurvedic practices like oiling, cleansing, and detoxifying keep us balanced and healthy all year.

- **Conclusion: Dance with the Seasons.**

The basic principle of Ayurveda is to be in tune and synchronized with Mother Nature. Ritucharya is a seasonal routine where lifestyle, diet, and habits are incorporated according to all seasons of shifting energies. When this finds space within your life, you will not find it difficult when the whole year comes into your being and treads with ease and balance.

As seasons come, we must come, too. Our bodies simply reflect what's going on around us. If we can adjust our habits to flow like water and work according to the earth's natural cycles, we will be in balance, prevent disease, and be more in tune with the planet. Life becomes a dance, and we think only to move with the beat of seasons and always be in step with nature's song.

Only by following dharma can true happiness and success be achieved. Dharma is how one can realize one's life or professional work aim. Dharma helps to better one's entirety and brings peace of mind. Kindness, generosity, and restraint over one's speech and thoughts must also be practiced. Constant reflection is a must, and time needs to be dedicated to reflecting on how those thoughts may influence action or whether one can continue to be the best that one can be.

Chapter 11: The Power of Restraint – Suppressible and Unsuppressible Urges

We live in the middle of thousands of emotional and physical impulses occurring in our day. Some merely pass through like a fleeting thought within the head; others are authoritarian desires, and many can lead us into our behaviors if only we give them entrance. Ayurveda recognizes this power of urges but teaches the art of discrimination- knowing when to suppress and let them run their course. This understanding of urges' equilibrium is one's pathway to health on both the mind and body levels.

Understanding Suppressible and Unsuppressible Urges

Ayurveda categorized desires into two forms, mainly those that are suppressible and those that can freely be expressed for our good. Typically, suppressible desires resonate with behaviours that can hurt us psychologically, emotionally, or socially. Conversely, unsuppressible desires are those that are natural body functions and, when suppressed, cause body discomfort and health issues.

Let us begin with suppressible desires. These are emotional responses such as anger, jealousy, fear, and impulses connected with language, like speaking abusively or gossiping, or related to the body, such as stealing and violence. Imagine you are working in a workplace where everyone has been waiting patiently for a promotion that another colleague is getting. The initial response would have been feelings of jealousy and the urge to speak about these concerns to another individual about how unfair everything was. Ayurveda teaches that these urges, natural as they are, need to be suppressed. Controlling the urge to condemn or engage in negative emotion helps protect personal mental hygiene and relations.

However, there are some compulsions that no man can suppress. Think of hunger, thirst, tears, flatulence, sleep, seminal discharge, yawning, and sneezing-they're your way of keeping the balance right and must not be suppressed lest it gets uncomfortable or even ailing. You could have experienced a brief headache or a heavy head the last time you suppressed a sneeze. According to Ayurveda, such urges serve a purpose and should be allowed to happen naturally since they do their bit of maintaining physical balance, too.

Balancing Emotional and Physical Urges

The only way to control impulses is not by pretending they do not exist but by taking control. The ability to recognize such emotional impulses the moment they arise could empower one to take charge of the reaction. For example, anger can be best responded to by stepping away, taking deep breaths, and letting it peak before forcing it down. Such control may prevent potential damage and leave one in peace of mind.

Likewise, reservations about speaking-related impulses like gossiping or interrupting improve rapport among people. After all, there is a need to vent some anger and share secrets, but the above acts usually lead to remorse and miscommunications. The better someone can refrain from such impulses, the more others will trust them and restore accord at work and personal levels.

The first lesson that Ayurveda teaches us is the answer to listening to body signals, particularly physical urges, such as unsuppressible ones, such as hunger and thirst. If one allows hunger for too long, the digestive fire or Agni gets weakened, leading to fatigue and irritability. Similarly, holding a sneeze leads to discomfort and more severe health complications, such as headaches or respiratory issues. Respecting these natural urges is a form of respecting the body's wisdom.

Another place where balance needs to be exercised relates to exercise. Ayurveda says one should not exercise after eating because working out on a full tummy stirs up Kapha. Utilized at the right time and in adequate amounts, exercise entails a host of benefits: it lightens the body, facilitates digestion, gives energy, and causes a lessening of aging. On the other hand, too much of this has adverse effects, including excessive thirst, weakening of the body, and weakening of the dhatus. Thus, the correct mechanism lies in that balance with a refreshing yet not distressing routine.

Balancing through Self-Control

It is not just taming evil impulses but liberation from an unhealthy practice. Ayurveda propitiates the unique gradual method of quitting addictions or hurtful habits called Vriddhi-Kshaya. This method is about the smooth transition from unhealthy behaviors into healthy choices over time, thus making it more accessible.

For example, if you wish to give up smoking, Ayurveda suggests tapering off gradually: on the first day, for example, drop three-quarters of the regular dosage, halve that for two days, and less by the end of a week. This has adapted your body more normally and does not let the withdrawal symptoms jolt in with their attendant intense cravings. This mode of dealing with the stressors decreases stress but at the same time develops self-discipline in the long run.

Charak's teachings, in his nutshell version, says control does not mean to deprive. Proper well-being must control one's enjoyment of oneself. When a point is realized, where some emotional or physical urge comes as a signal that needs to be attended to has been crossed, that is the best time for self-control. Kindness, gentleness, and patience about oneself are what self-control is. It is a balance and not a deprivation of pleasure and spontaneity.

Conclusion: The Art of Restraint

It is how we learn to dance with our urgings and determine which to fulfill and which to restrain; it is a path to inner peace and physical wellness. In this vein, Ayurveda teaches that health isn't when one isn't sick but an evolving state of balance between mind, body, and spirit. We cultivate this balance by discerning which urgings to suppress and which to honor.

Living under restraint, especially in a society geared more toward instant gratification, is an excellent way of connecting to ourselves at the level of our deeper selves. When we take the time to listen to our bodies, honor what our emotions tell us to do, and be aware of our actions, we add not only to our well-being but to alignment with some natural balance, characteristic of life. This finally brings us toward an easier way of being, pursuing our development, and cultivating each other better.

Chapter 12: The Vital Energies of Exercise

For most of us, exercise is a tool for staying fit. In Ayurveda, the meaning is much more profound: physical activity becomes a means for generating and maintaining Prana, that energy source in our body that makes us alive, makes us live, and makes us vital. If one exercises according to a particular constitution or dosha, then it's something more than an ordinary routine; instead, it's a practice where the body and mind are nourished and cultivated. With this Ayurvedic view of exercise, we come to learn how to use our strength and endurance while at the same time improving our health and well-being.

Benefits of Exercise in Ayurveda

If done correctly, well-practiced yoga, as taught by Ayurveda, is one of the most potent weapons for health and long life. It's a movement that helps stimulate the Agni or digestive fire, removes toxins, and leaves a person feeling light and clear. That is why you'll feel this energy after a good workout, as though a weight has been lifted off your shoulders.

Exercise bears profound benefits upon the doshas as well. While Kaphas feel excessive lethargy or are being weighed down, exercise will stimulate those with this constitution to awaken their bodies and minds. Pitta type naturally contains more energy, but due to overheating or irritation, moderate amounts of exercise help release pent-up energy in a balanced manner. Gentle, rhythmic movement provides a sense of grounding and stabilization in Vata persons, who are primarily restless or anxious. Consider the case of Raj, a thirty-something-year-old who began running every morning after years of a sedentary lifestyle. In the initial phase, it was a hard push; he would tire quickly and feel heavy in the legs. With time, as his endurance built up, he felt more energetic throughout the day and more concentrated and less stressed. "Running not only turned out to be a physical sport for Raj but was also a way of mentally refreshing himself and his mind amidst the chaos." Such an effect is not surprising in Ayurveda. Exercise conditions the body sharpens the mind, and strengthens emotional hardiness.

Exercises by Doshas

Ayurveda doesn't believe in a size fits all exercise routine. Instead, everyone is advised to choose their own according to dosha. Here is the breakdown of exercises suitable for each dosha:

- Vata Dosha: Vatas are inherently energetic but can sometimes be unpredictable. Ayurveda anchors doshas with slow, steady movement, and the grounding process is achieved through yoga, Tai Chi, or brisk walking. Thus, Vatas are kept grounded and less flighty by steadily steadying their often roving minds.
- Pitta Dosha: Essentially competitive and intense personalities who naturally desire to succeed. But excess inner heat burns them out or irritates them. Pitta dosha people will find merit in cooling and not-too-heavy activities like swimming, cycling, or hiking, as they give off energy without overheating the person or becoming overly aggressive.
- Kapha Dosha: Kaphas are heavy-bodied and strong but can become lazy if they do not engage in activities. Ayurveda recommends energizing activities that boost the body and

break stagnation. Running, dancing, or aerobics are also suitable for kaphas since they increase blood flow and keep the mind active.

The exercises individuals choose should resonate genuinely with their dosha; they'll enjoy it more and find it a breeze to maintain their routine. An anxious Vata might find solace in slow, mindful yoga movements, while a Kapha, feeling weighed down, might be invigorated by the fast rhythm of a dance class. You're working with your natural tendencies instead of fighting them.

Natural Strength and Physical Endurance

In Ayurveda, Bala, or natural strength, is a quality each of us possesses to greater or lesser degrees. Strength is more than muscle; it extends to stamina, immunity, and resilience. Some have innate Bala and seem as strong as an ox, while others must nurse it. In any case, Ayurveda offers everyone the opportunity to develop strength and endurance if approached in a well-rounded program.

Let's return to Raj, the man who found solace in running. Time crept past as he continued his daily run in the morning and realized that stamina did not develop- not just outside it, too. He acquired even more tolerance at work, more flexibility towards life's setbacks, and even created a sense of discipline. Bala, in a nutshell, when we boost our natural power through regular exercise, it has implications for the mind and how we deal with life.

Ayurveda says that steadiness and moderation are the keys to endurance. Exercise by your natural biorhythm, when you have maximum energy and feel best at dawn, allows you to tap into your natural power of strength. On the other hand, overexertion wastes your energy and knocks out your doshas, leaving you smelling of fatigue, thirst, or injury. Ayurveda teaches us to listen to and appreciate our bodies—to know when to push on and when to rest.

Exercise has tremendous benefits that transcend the body. It builds Ojas, i.e., energies that protect against diseases and bad moods. An exercise schedule gives a person a feeling of lightness, power, and readiness for any event. If taken consciously, exercise is not just something that helps us develop physical fitness but also a road to mental clarity and inner peace.

Conclusion:

According to Ayurveda, any body movement is a Life-Giving Exercise. This means that the pursuit of a fit body must include more than the achievement of fitness; it is the art of keeping the body balanced with mind and spirit and creating movement and nourishment for the flow of Prana and the growth of our natural resilience." As you begin to do activities that flow in sync with your dosha, you can develop your style of movement, which is full of balance and glee.

Whether it is a run in the morning, evening yoga practice, or a swim over the weekend, the idea is to invite some degree of activity into your body that would feel right and comfortable. Exercise never has to be a chore; it could instead be a celebration of the human body's possibilities that lead someone to deep well-being. It's precisely then that we enter rhythm with our body's energy, and the true power of exercise is unlocked: building us into more than just physically strong people who hold that energy and sense of vitality long after the practice.

Chapter 14: The Science of Eating - Ayurveda and Diet

Ayurveda considers food a source of nutrition and vital energy that feeds the body, mind, and soul. Still, all such benefits depend on our Agni (digestive fire) and Prakriti (constitution) interaction. Thus, keeping the secrets of Ayurvedic health in these two elements, tailoring diet according to individual needs, unravels the true potential of food as medicine.

Agni: The Digestive Fire

Imagine a fire burning inside you that breaks down what you eat, converting it into energy and nourishment. This is Agni, or digestive fire, central to Ayurveda. If your Agni burns brightly, you feel invigorated, and with smooth digestion, your body absorbs the nutrients. But if you have sloppy Agni, you become sluggish and bloated, and even toxins gather- to, say, Ama.

Ayurveda describes four types of Agni:

- Sama Agni: (Balanced Fire) It is the ideal state. In this state, digestion becomes smooth, and all types of food can digest. Usually, individuals possessing Agni in a balanced state are well. Vishama Agni (Irregular Fire) is a normal condition in the patient with Vata, which makes Agni variable causing spastic digestion, gas, and distension.

- Tikshna Agni: This is the kind of Agni typically identified in Pitta types due to being too hot, causing rapid digestion that leads to heartburn and hunger pangs.
- Manda Agni: This is the Agni characteristic mostly found among Kapha types due to a more gentle weakness with heaviness, dullness, and weight gain.
- Ayurvedic nutrition involves finding your Agni and aligning your diet to balance it. Warm food grounding will do the trick if you have Vishama Agni. Excellent food soothing is a golden piece of advice for Tikshna Agni.

Diet Prescriptions Based on Doshas

Your Prakriti is the balance of three doshas- Vata, Pitta, and Kapha - in you. The dietary requirements of each of these different aspects are unique to make sure there is balance once again. Alright, let's get into it in detail:

Diet for Vata Dosha

Vata types are inherently light, dry, and cold. Therefore, they require warming, nourishing, and grounding foods.

- Recommended Foods include root vegetables, cooked grain such as rice and oats, ghee, nuts, and warming spices like cinnamon and ginger.
- Avoid cold drinks, raw salads, and dry foods such as crackers or popcorn, as those irritate Vata.

- Food Recommendations: Eat smaller portions more often, and don't skip meals. Irregular food habits can imbalance Vata

Diet for Pitta Dosha

Pittas are those with hot bodies and fiery temperaments who love having cooling, refreshing, and soothing foods.

- Some recommended food items in this category are sweet fruits like melons and pears, cooling dairy, green leafy vegetables, and coconut water.
- Shun hot, sour, salty things, fried or fermented, foods- everything stimulates inflammation by sustaining Pitta.
- Food Suggestions: Leniently flavor foods and avoid overeating as it may trigger digestive fires.

Diet for Kapha Dosha

The Kaphas are fat, slow, and moist, requiring a light, warm, and stimulating diet.

- Fruits and foodstuffs that should be suggested include barley, millet, beans, bitter vegetables such as bitter gourd and methi leaves, and warming spices such as pepper and turmeric.
- To be avoided are sweet, oily, and cold foodstuffs like ice cream heavy sweets, which enhance Kaphas' slowness.

- Food Recommendations: Because digestion is slower, dinner needs to be eaten earlier in the evening. Additionally, there should be sufficient time between meals.

Light Food　　Heavy Food

/\　　/\

Air Fire　　Earth Water

Ayurvedic Diet Principles

A person should eat according to his Agni. What he eats is to digest without giving him discomfort. Light food, with the predominance of air and fire elements, stimulates Agni and causes lesser damage, even when consumed in larger quantities. Heavy food, with earth and water elements, does not stimulate Agni, as their qualities are against the promotion of Agni, which may be used in excess. Ayurveda states that heavier foods should not fill more than ½ or 1/3rd of capacity, and even the lightest foods should not be so filling that they can't get space in the stomach. Consuming excessive amounts, regardless of the food, damages Agni. Therefore, it should be taken only till satiation called Tripti. People with a more vital metabolism and exercise properly can digest more strongly. Moreover, intake after finishing the consumables of a meal suppresses Agni and deranges metabolism. The points mentioned above demonstrate why eating should be mindful and how appropriate time slots of consumption will reward individuals.

The following principles ensure that one's diet harmonizes with Ayurvedic consciousness.

- Fresh and Seasonal Foods: Fresh, local, and in-season foods are more likely to help your natural balance and are easier to digest.
- All Six Tastes: Ayurveda recognizes six tastes: sweet, sour, salty, bitter, pungent, and astringent. A balanced meal must include all six to handle every aspect of digestion and nourishment. For example, sweet rice gives energy, while bitter greens detoxify.
- Do Not Overindulge. Ayurveda advises stopping eating when you feel you have satisfied your hunger by 75%. If you overfeed, you load too much of a burden on Agni. This weakens Agni, leading to Ama, or indigestion.
- Conscious Ingestion of Nourishment: Nourishment should be taken with focused time without the temptations of television or your cell phone; this allows your body to break down your food better.
- Eating to the Clock: The heaviest meal should be consumed around midday when Agni is at its peak. A light but nourishing breakfast and a light dinner should ensure that all eating is completed by early evening and that the digestion process is complete before sleep.
- Drink Water: Drink enough water, though Ayurveda advises sipping warm water while eating and avoiding cold drinks as they cool Agni.

Conclusion: Food as Medicine

Food is the most reachable medicine. The knowledge of your Agni and Prakriti will help you determine a diet that matches your dosha, transform your approach toward nourishing your body and mind, and bring more to life than just being an instrument for mere survival-the balance, aliveness, and goodness for the rest of the aspects of life.

At your Chronic Fatiguef: Am I nourishing my body in alignment with its natural desire? Aligning diet with the wisdom of Ayurveda means having food have the power it was meant to have: the power to heal, energize, and sustain. This is related to respecting and becoming a friend to what you eat rather than deprivation.

Chapter 15: The Six Tastes of Life

Ayurveda understands that taste is more than a flash on the tongue. Taste has a powerful influence on our health and balance of life. The six tastes, sweet (Madhur), sour (amla), salty (lavan), bitter (tikta), pungent (katu), and astringent (kashay), compose a general structure for understanding how food influences the body, mind, and spirit. When these tastes are balanced in the diet, we are better aligned with the doshas and have overall long-term wellness.

According to the Ayurvedic sage Charak, rasa is the essence that is perceived by the tongue. Taste is perceived as an interaction of mahabhootas, a combination of water and earth. Water is the universal element deeply inherent in taste perception between water and earth. However, each taste has a particular arrangement of components that decides the qualities and results.

Six Tastes and Their Impact on Doshas

Each of the six tastes has specific properties that combine either harmoniously with Vata, Pitta, and Kapha or occasionally in disharmony with them, balancing and, at other times, aggravating. This insight will enable us to fashion the diet we need.

1. Sweet (Madhur)

Mahabhootas: Water, Earth

Effects: The sweet taste is nourishing and cooling; it retains strength, immunity, and vitality

Balances: Vata and Pitta

Aggravates: Kapha

Examples: Banana and mango, rice and wheat, milk, ghee and honey, and jaggery.

The sweet taste is pleasing and soothing. It calms the fears of Vata individuals and decreases Pitta heat, but a surplus adds up Kapha, making one gain weight and lazy.

2. Sour (Amla)

Mahabhootas: Earth, Fire

Effects: The sour food energizes and stimulates digestion, but it heats the body.

Balances: Vata

Aggravates: Pitta and Kapha

Examples: Oranges, yogurt, pickles, and tamarind.

Sour sharpens the mind and senses and stimulates appetite, salivation, and metabolism. It is helpful for Vata, but its warmth troubles Pitta, causing hair greying and falling, weakening tendons, and making Kapha heavier.

3. Salty (Lavan)

Mahabhootas: Water, Fire

Effects: Salty foods tend to ground, flavor, digest, and hydrate.

Balances: Vata

Aggravates: Pitta and Kapha

Examples: Sea salt, rock salt, and salty snacks.

The quality of salt grounds Vata, but too much salt irritates Pitta and causes edema due to excess Kapha.

4. Bitter (Tikta)

Mahabhootas: Air, Fire

Effects: Bitter foods purify, cool, clean the blood, and help clear the mind.

Balances: Pitta and Kapha

Aggravates: Vata

Examples: Bitter melon, neem, turmeric, kale, and spinach.

The bitter taste is for purification. It is a good antidote when Pitta and Kapha accumulate. Tikta removes itching, burning, and extra watery, slimy mucus from the body. But its lightness can negatively impact Vata, causing extreme dryness.

5. Pungent (Katu)

Mahabhootas: Air, Space

Effects: Pungent food is a warming and stimulating food that stimulates flow and metabolism.

Balances: Kapha

Aggravates: Vata and Pitta

Examples: Spices like ginger, garlic, black pepper, and chili.

Pungent food wakes the body up, induces appetite, and heals wounds just as the Kapha needs, but its force disturbs the balance of the pitta's fire and vata's moisture, causing infertility or needle-like pain.

6. Astringent (Kashay)

Mahabhootas: Air, Earth

Effects: Astringent flavors are dry and cool, decrease inflammation, and have an overall cleaning effect.

Balances: Pitta and Kapha

Aggravates: Vata

Examples: legumes, green bananas, pomegranates, and herbs like turmeric and fenugreek.

Due to their binding action, astringents tone and tighten the tissues. They are soothing to Pitta and Kapha, but drying can irritate Vata, causing bloating and a lack of skin tone.

Taste	Elements	Balances	Aggravates
Sweet	Water, Earth	Vata, Pitta	Kapha
Sour	Earth, Fire	Vata	Kapha, Pitta
Salty	Water, Fire	Vata	Kapha, Pitta
Bitter	Air, Fire	Kapha	Pitta, Vata
Pungent	Air, Space	Pitta, Kapha	Vata
Astringent	Air, Earth	Pitta, Kapha	Vata

Balancing Tastes for Optimal Health

Ayurveda advises using all six tastes in the perfect diet in every meal. Each taste must make a specific input, and a mix ensures balanced nutrition. For instance:

The Vata type would require the addition of sweetness, acidity, and saltiness to stabilize the aggravation of Vata.

The Pitta type would benefit by including a mix of sweetness, bitterness, and astringency to cool down their inflamed nature.

The flavor that would overcome heaviness and rekindle the metabolism in a Kapha person should be bitter, pungent, and astringent.

Take Riya, a Pitta type who complained of acid reflux. She changed her diet to include cooling and bitter foods, such as leafy greens, buttermilk, and cucumbers and avoided spicy or sour tastes. She felt the change. This small change made a big difference to her mood and energy level.

Add The Six Tastes To Your Daily Cooking

Adding the six tastes to your everyday dishes is easy. Here are some general tips:

- Base: Sweet grains like rice or wheat are used mainly as the base.
- Layer on the dishes: Add some sourness, like lemon juice, saltiness, sea salt, and bitterness, like fenugreek or spinach leaves.
- Equilibrium with Spice: The Pitta types must avoid ginger and black pepper.
- Finish with Astringents: Legumes or astringent fruits like pomegranate seeds can add the final touch to a well-rounded meal.

A simple khichdi rice and lentil porridge balances the five flavors: sweet rice, salty rock salt, a dash of lemon, a hint of pungent ginger, a sprinkling of turmeric, and lentils, which are astringent.

Conclusion:

In Ayurveda, six tastes offer more than flavors -they are the pathway to balance and health. A look into how each impacts the doshas and how they can be incorporated into one's diet may advance the natural rhythm of life.

So the next time you sit at the dining table, take your time and enjoy every taste, knowing that each of those bites is an opportunity to create harmony within.

Chapter 16: How to Detoxify the Body – The Concept of Aama/Ajirna

“Good health," says Ayurveda, "is not just the absence of disease but rather the presence of a harmonious body and mind accompanied by the removal of toxins." In other words, undigested food toxins accumulate in the body when this balance is disrupted. Here, then, follows discomfort and illness. Therefore, it is a vital learning step toward preserving vitality and harmony to understand what Aama is: toxins in the body.

Understanding Aama – Toxins in the Body

Aama means "unripe" or "undigested." It is the stuff resulting from the digestive system's incomplete or wrong processing function. Imagine it like a sticky, poisonous sludge plugged into the natural flow in your body, preventing nutrients from being absorbed and waste from being removed.

Aama is typically linked to an imbalance of Kapha, which manifests in the system as heaviness, excessive salivation, restlessness, and slowness. If left unchecked, Aama will engage Pitta, which manifests as inflammation, acidic and sour burping, and burning sensations. It can become severe and cause dizziness. The presence of Aama is a sign of slow digestive fire, low Agni, and the body calling for a reboot.

Causes and Symptoms of Aama Buildup

Causes for the Formation of Aama

Aama may occur because of unhygienic food habits, lifestyle disorders, or emotional disturbances.

Common reasons:

- **Dietary Causes**: Overeating, consuming stale or contaminated food, eating raw, heavy, or too dry food, or experiencing very hot or cold temperatures can weaken digestion.
- **Lifestyle Causes:** The same may occur due to irregular eating times, ignoring meals, or eating distractedly; watching TV or looking at your phone can weaken Agni.
- **Emotional Causes:** Negative emotions, such as sadness, anger, jealousy, or fear, can dominate during meals and weaken digestion. Even where you eat is a factor because if you feel rushed or stressed while eating, Aama most definitely forms.

Symptoms of Aama

When Aama starts forming, your body sends some clear signals. Getting to know the symptoms is the first move toward the solution:

Physically, it presents with bloating of the abdomen and body, swelling in the cheeks and eyes, abdominal pain, and a collection of stool, urine, or gas.

It produces burning sensations, dizziness, and excessive thirst due to Pitta's involvement.

Chronic conditions will arise if these signs are overlooked because toxins spread across the body's systems.

Detoxification Techniques in Ayurveda

The Ayurveda view of detoxing is not about being on a crash diet or starving your body but balancing your digestive system without any strain to remove Aama. This is how you can start:

1. Diet Changes

- Fasting or Intermittent Fasting: Even a short fast can reinstall your digestive system. If you cannot fast, eat light, easily digestible foods such as soups or khichdi-a, a rice and lentil porridge mixture.
- Detoxifying Foods: Include fruit and vegetable juices like orange, carrot, beetroot, and celery juice for digestive benefits and to cleanse the system. Other drinks like ginger tea can kindle Agni and help break down toxins.
- Avoid Triggers: While detoxing, one should avoid fried or stale food and focus on clean, warm, fresh food.

2. Warm Pressure

Applying warm temperatures to the abdomen reduces bloating and promotes easier digestion. A warm pad or heating pad over the abdominal area stimulates Agni and counteracts the heaviness caused by Kapha.

3. Ayurvedic Therapies

When Aama is quite strong, it is recommended that Vaman (induced vomiting) or Virechan (purgation) be performed as part of treatment to flush the digestive system.

Ayurvedic Way of Eating

Detoxification involves not only what you eat but also how you eat it. Ayurveda cultivates mindful eating practices that help you digest and avoid the aggregation of unnecessary toxins.

- Eat on Time: Eat at set times to maintain the regular digestive fire.
- Sit and experience: Sit down to eat in quiet, serene surroundings without radio, television, or cell phone ringing. Eating should be an opportunity to reconnect with food, the body, and loved ones.
- Eat mindfully: Chew slowly and taste each bite. Eating too quickly will overwhelm digestion, and eating too slowly will dull one's Agni.

- Cleanliness Exercise: Always wash your hands and face before meals. This simple hygienic act prepares your body and mind for nourishment.
- Be Present: Do not condemn or criticize others in front of the people sitting with you while eating. Peace and happiness facilitate digestion.
- Listen to Your Hunger: Start eating when you feel too hungry, and stop when you're 75% full. Overeating is a direct invitation for Aama.

Conclusion: Restoring Balance Through Awareness

Aama formation is a significant pointer in that the body is out of alignment but can be detoxified and rejuvenated through simple changes in the mindset to diet and lifestyle and reignite Agni, thus bringing balance back into the system. Knowing the signs and the possible causes of the toxin build-up gives one the power to prevent it before it takes its toll on health.

Let food and eating be a ritual. Enjoy your food with respect and consciousness because every bite can heal or hurt your body.

Chapter 17: Incompatible Diets

Ayurveda does not consider food merely food—it is a means of balancing the body and mind. Any diet that imbalances vata, pitta, and Kapha but does not remove the imbalanced doshas is called an incompatible diet. Incorrect food combinations cause disorders in the digestive system, producing toxins such as Aama, as discussed previously. This causes further derangement of the doshas. Ayurveda explains Viruddha Ahara or incompatible diets, and how careful eating habits support us in maintaining balance and health. Purification therapies like Vaman (therapeutic vomiting) and Virechan (therapeutic purgation), or herbs that calm imbalanced doshas, are essential for detoxification and dosha balancing.

Food Incompatibility: Detection and Avoidance

Food incompatibility refers to mixes that are excellent in their own right but become poisonous upon being mixed and consumed. The mixes cause undue perplexity or overwhelm the digestive fire or Agni, where toxin formations occur. Examples are:

- **Milk and Sour Fruit:** The acidity of sour fruits curdles milk, spoiling the digesting process and producing bloating or gas.
- **Honey and Boiling Water:** Heating changes the chemical properties of honey and makes it dangerous to ingest.
- **Fish and Milk** are heavy foods with conflicting properties. When mixed, they often lead to skin disorders and dosha imbalances.

- **Cold Drinks with Meals:** Cold beverages extinguish Agni, slowing digestion and causing toxin buildup.

To maintain equilibrium, avoid these combinations and consume foods that match your dosha and digestive capacity.

Four types of dietetic incompatibility

According to Sage Charak, there are specific factors that contribute to dietetic incompatibilities, which disrupt digestion and lead to the formation of toxins (Aama). These incompatibilities are categorized based on geography, season, digestive fire, and doshas. Additionally, incompatibilities can arise from improper food properties, sequences, combinations, personal preferences, and rituals. Here's a detailed look at these types:

1. Incompatibility According to Geography

The environment in which an individual lives plays a crucial role in determining appropriate dietary choices.

- Those living in desert or dry regions should avoid very dry or excessively spicy foods, as these can exacerbate dryness and heat in the body.
- Conversely, individuals in humid climates should refrain from consuming overly cold foods, which can disrupt digestion and promote Kapha imbalance.

2. Incompatibility According to Season

Seasonal changes influence the body's doshas, and diet should adapt accordingly.

- **Winter**: Avoid cold and dry foods or herbs, as they aggravate Vata and dampen Agni.
- **Summer**: Refrain from consuming warm, pungent, and bitter foods, as they can intensify Pitta. Aligning diet with seasonal needs helps maintain dosha balance and prevents digestive disturbances.

3. Incompatibility According to Digestive Fire (Agni)

Agni, or digestive fire, varies among individuals and should guide food intake:

- Those with a strong appetite should not be underfed, as insufficient food leaves their digestive fire unutilized, potentially causing weakness or toxin buildup.
- Those with a weakened appetite should avoid overeating, as this overwhelms their Agni, leading to indigestion and toxin formation.

4. Incompatibility According to Doshas

This occurs when foods or herbs with properties similar to a dosha are consumed in excess, causing an imbalance:

- **Vata**: Consuming dry, cold, or light foods can aggravate Vata.

- **Pitta**: Overindulgence in hot, spicy, or sour foods can intensify.
- **Kapha**: Eating heavy, oily, or sweet foods can increase Kapha's sluggishness.

Other Types of Incompatibilities

In addition to the four main categories, there are other incompatibilities that Ayurveda highlights:

1. **Incompatibility According to Property**: Combining foods with opposing properties, like hot and cold, can disrupt digestion.
2. **Incompatibility According to Sequence**: Eating meals before the body is ready—such as when it feels hungry or passes stool and urine—can lead to digestive issues.
3. **Incompatibility According to Combination**: Specific food pairings, such as milk with sour or salty foods, are inherently incompatible and can cause a buildup of toxins.
4. **Incompatibility According to Liking**: Eating foods that you dislike or do not feel pleasant can negatively affect your mental and digestive health.
5. **Incompatibility According to Ritual**: Meals should be consumed in a quiet and peaceful environment. Eating in a chaotic or stressful setting can disrupt digestion and impact dosha balance.

Health Problems Due to Incompatible Food Combinations

Unsuitable diets lead to a set of short-term and long-term health disorders. The immediate reactions include bloating, indigestion, nausea, and acid reflux. Long-term causes include dosha imbalances and chronic conditions such as:

- **Kapha Aggravation:** Slows down Agni, congestion, respiratory disorders, or obesity
- **Pitta Aggravation:** Inflammation, acidity, herpes, psoriasis, vitiligo, eczema, or other skin issues
- **Vata Aggravation:** Lack of strength, intelligence, memory, unbalanced digestion, joint pain.

These issues occur due to the backup of Aama, a sticky substance of undigested food that clogs the channels and breaks down the functioning.

How to overcome the chronic effects of an incompatible diet

When Aama piles up, cleaning has to be done to reassess the balance. Ayurveda offers cleansing through diet, lifestyle, and medicated therapies -

Diet and Lifestyle Adjustments:

- **Light Food Diet:** Switch to easily digestible foods, soups, or khichdi, a rice-lentil porridge.

- **Fruit Juices and Herbal Teas:** Lemon water, orange juice, or ginger tea stimulate digestion and help detoxify.
- **Intermittent Fasting:** Fasting or a small intake would reset the digestive fire and burn all the toxins.
- **Exercise**: Stimulating metabolism through exercise can assist in getting rid of the Aama.

Vaman (Therapeutic Vomiting)

Vaman is an Ayurveda-controlled cleaning therapy intended to remove toxins resulting from Kapha from the upper digestive system. This treatment is most effective in conditions caused by Kapha's aggravation, such as excess mucus, heaviness, or nausea. In the hands of an Ayurvedic practitioner, Vaman can cleanse toxins and reactivate Agni for a lighter, better-balanced body.

Virechan (Therapeutic Purgation)

Virechan is a simple, purgative therapy that helps remove Pitta-toxin residues from the lower intestines. It is beneficial for treating diseases such as acidity, inflammation, and skin disorders. Virechan reinstates digestive health by purifying the colon and the liver, thereby balancing Pitta.

If done correctly, these therapies guarantee complete purification without further accumulation of Aama.

Guidelines to Assure Safety in Food Combinations

Ayurveda provides excellent guidelines about not combining foods and encourages proper digestion.

- **Do Not Combine Heavily Prepared Foods:** Never combine two heavy foods, like cheese and fried food, as this will strain your digestive process.
- **Freshly Cooked Food:** Eating newly prepared foods less burdens the body than stale or reheated food.
- **Intake of Ice Foods:** Ingestion of icy or raw foods in excessive amounts reduces Agni.
- **Simple Foods:** Digestion can be effortlessly maintained by combining complementary tastes rather than excessively complicated dishes.
- **Time:** Eat at proper times so that the stomach is clean and empty before the next meal.
- **Eating Awareness:** Do not eat while using a telephone or television, but slowly and rightly chew the food.

Herbal Teas for Everyday Ailments:

There is nothing easier than herbal teas to enhance digestion and dosha balance. Here are just a few authentic Ayurvedic preparations for everyday conditions:

- **Digestive Tea:** Ginger, fennel, and cumin enhance Agni, alleviate bloating, and digest the food.

- **Detox Tea:** Turmeric, coriander, and mint tea cleanse the liver and decrease Ama.
- **Calming Tea:** Chamomile and licorice tea soothes Vata, giving relief and refreshing sleep.
- **Kapha Balancing Tea:** Black pepper, tulsi, and dry ginger reduce stagnation and sluggishness.

These teas complement detoxing practices like Vaman and Virechan for a balanced digestive system.

Take the case of Lisa, a marketing executive aged 32 years who had suffered from chronic bloating, acid reflux, and tiredness because of her irregular eating patterns and fondness for trying out various cuisines. A dinner party that had grilled fish with a dash of lemon, a yogurt dip, and chilled soda increased her symptoms to extreme abdominal pain. She sought help from an Ayurveda doctor, who introduced her to Viruddha Ahara, or incompatible diets. Her diet had mixed fish and dairy, sour food, and carbonated drinks that messed up her digestive fire (Agni) and produced toxins (Aama). Moreover, her hurried, inattentive nature of eating had compounded the matter.

The practitioner gave her a gentle detoxification plan, Virechan (purgation therapy) to cleanse her system, dietary adjustments to avoid incompatible combinations, herbal teas like ginger-fennel-cumin for digestion, and mindful eating practices. In weeks, Lisa's symptoms improved dramatically. Her experience underscored the importance of aligning dietary habits with Ayurvedic principles, transforming her approach to food from convenience-driven to mindful and intentional, paving the way for better health and balance.

Conclusion: Eating with Awareness

The unique Ayurvedic principle of incompatible diets teaches us that even healthy foods may harm when put together incorrectly. So, understand which food combinations may harm and alter your dietary habits. Introduce detox therapies such as Vaman and Virechan to re-establish balance and energy within oneself.

Let your meals nourish your body, mind, and soul by embracing the concept of an incompatible diet.

Chapter 18: The Formulations of Ayurveda

The healing tradition of Ayurveda is rich in its diversified formulations, designed to illuminate the therapeutic power of herbs. From pastes to herbal powders and teas, all these preparations find their roots in natural balance and can be individualized for different ailments. Understanding the forms and their uses is the key to better grasping how Ayurveda offers a holistic approach to health and wellness.

Types of Ayurvedic Medicine

1. Herbal Decoction Tea (Kashaya/Kvath)

A decoction is a light, potent remedy made from herbs boiled in water or milk to extract their active properties. It is also known as herbal tea. Add honey or ghee to the herbal tea. Teas are discussed in detail in the next chapter.

- Preparation: Mix one teaspoon of dry powdered herb with four times as much water, for example, 60 ml. Boil on medium heat until the water is reduced to 1/8th. Pour and drink while still warm. Do not cover the pan while boiling to make the decoction light.
- Examples:

Digestive tea: ginger, black pepper, and cumin. Anti-fatigue tea: dates and raisins.

Rejuvenating tea: Guduchi, haritaki, and shatavari.

Weight reducing tea: Nagarmotha, turmeric, and kutki.

- Usage: Herbal tea can stimulate digestion, increase energy, or treat particular conditions depending on the herbs.

2. Pastes (Kalka)

A paste is a semi-fluid preparation of ground wet or dry herbs with water or milk. It can be applied locally or even taken orally for specific objectives.

- Preparation: Grind fresh herbs such as coriander or mint with a small amount of water. Dry herbs need to be mixed with three teaspoons of water before grinding.
- Examples: Paste of ginger and garlic for detoxification; coriander paste for cooling effects.
- Usage: Pastes are versatile. They can be used as poultices for skin conditions or ingested for internal imbalances.

3. Herbal Powders (Churna)

Churna are finely powdered herbs that may be combined to form a specific treatment. They are amongst the easiest and most variable forms of Ayurvedic preparations.

- Preparation: Herbs can be dried, powdered finely, and stored in close containers.
- Examples: Triphala powder, haritaki-bibhitaki-amalaki for digestive purposes, and turmeric powder for anti-inflammatory action.

- Usage: Powders can be taken orally with lukewarm water, honey, or ghee or added to decoctions.

Preparation Techniques and Uses

Ayurvedic formulations rely on ancient techniques and some modern styles that help in getting the greatest possible potency of herbs:

- Expressed Juices (Savarasa): Fresh herbs are crushed, or dry herbs are soaked in twice the amount of water to squeeze out their juice. To express juice from dry herbs rather quickly, grind the dry herb and cook it eight times in water. When the mixture reduces to 1/4 of the original quantity, it can be used as a juice (2-4 ounces). These are used internally with rapid absorption and action, like enhancing immunity or controlling inflammation. Two drops of ghee or oil can be used with the juice for lubrication. Jaggery or salt can be used to modify the taste.
- Cold Infusions (Sheeta): Herbs are immersed in cool water overnight and strained. This method is useful for creating infusions of cooling herbs and is beneficial for Pitta imbalances.
- Hot Infusions (Fanta): These are the same as cold infusions, except the herb is soaked in warm water. Hot infusions are suitable for enhancing the potency of herbs.

Choosing the Appropriate Formulation to Administer for Treatment

The proper Ayurvedic preparation is selected depending on the dosha, the condition, and the objective of the treatment of the patient:

- For Vata Imbalances: Warm decoctions and pastes are grounding and soothing. Powders with ghee or milk increase nourishment.
- For Pitta Imbalances: Soothing preparations like cold infusions and tea with sandalwood and coriander cool off the heat excesses.
- For Kapha Imbalances: Stimulation decoctions with warming herbs like ginger and black pepper help reduce stagnation and heaviness.

Thus, Ayurveda offers customized and efficient treatments by matching its preparation with dosha.

Conclusion: Tapping into Ayurvedic Preparations

Ayurvedic preparations symbolize the philosophy of tailoring treatments according to individual requirements. Whether it is an alcoholic decoction to revitalize digestion, a cooling infusion to balance Pitta, or a herbal paste to treat inflammation, these preparations reflect the holistic approach that Ayurveda takes toward health. By learning to prepare and use these formulations, we could unlock the profound healing energy of this natural pharmacy.

Take time to implement these old practices daily and feel Ayurveda working its magic.

Chapter 19: Brews of Vitality: Herbal Teas for Every Need

Herbal teas, or kashaya, are a crucial aspect of Ayurveda, offering a healthy and capable solution for all our health and wellness concerns. These mixes of chosen herbs mean curing every disorder while keeping a person's well-being intact. With this knowledge of their preparations and functions, you can add these drinks to your routine and enjoy their remarkable curative properties.

Ayurvedic Herbal Teas Formulations

Ayurvedic herbal teas are made from herbs that resonate in tune with specific dosha imbalances or health-related problems. Some of the most essential tea formulations include the following:

1. Revitalising and Energizing Tea

- Ingredients: Jeevak, Rishbhak, Meda, Mahameda, Kakoli, Ksheerkakoli, Mung, Urad, Jeevanti, Licorice (Yastimadhu).
- Benefits: This tea refreshes the body and avoids muscular wasting. It provides energy to the body. As it contains water and earth elements, this tea is taken to build power.

2.Weight gaining Tea

- Ingredients: Ashwagandha, Bala, Vidarikand.
- Benefits: It develops muscle, promotes healthy weight gain, and provides general nutrition.

3. Weight Loss Tea

- Ingredients: Nagarmotha, Kustha, Turmeric, Vacha, Chitrak, Kutki.
- Benefits: Stretches the metabolism for weight gain. Its air and fire elements fuel Agni, which lowers Kapha.

4.Digestive Tea

- Ingredients: Chavya, Chitrak, Pippalimool, Ginger, Black Pepper, Pippali (Trikatu), Ajwain, Hing.
- Benefits: It stimulates digestive fire, reduces gas formation, and enhances appetite.

5.Complexion enhancing tea

- Ingredients: Sariva, Manjistha, Sandalwood (Chandan), Ushira, Licorice, Vidari, Durva, Naagkeshar.
- Benefits: Purify the blood and balance Bhrajak Pitta to regain the skin's natural glow.

6.Cardiac Health Tea

- Ingredients: Mango, Amlavetasa, Pomegranate, Aamda, Karaunda
- Benefits: Strengthens the heart and promotes cardiovascular health.

Benefits of Specific Herbal Blends

Each Ayurvedic tea is prepared with a specific intention, and that is to correct the dosha imbalance and obtain any of the following benefits:

- Anti-Fatigue Tea: Dates, Munakka, Raisins, Pomegranate, Figs, Sugarcane, and Rice Water.

This tea rejuvenates energy, fights fatigue, and strengthens the body's endurance.

- Anti-Burning Tea: Sandalwood, Anantmool, Ushira, Guduchi.

It cools the burning conditions in the body caused by Pitta, dispels burning sensations, and reduces inflammation.

- Anti-Itching Tea: Neem, Chandan, Jatamansi, Karanj, Kutaj, Sarshap, Yasti, Daruharidra, Nagarmotha.

This tea has anti-prickling properties and can cure skin irritation caused by allergies or dryness.

- Revitalizing Tea: Guduchi, Haritaki, Shatavari, Mandukparni, Punarnava, Jeevanti.

This tea rejuvenates the body and mind and increases life and strength.

- Anti-hemorrhoid Tea: Kutaj, Bael, Chitrak, Shuntha, Haritaki, Vacha, Daruhaldi. This tea resolves hemorrhoids and piles.
- Vitalizing Tea for Men: Jeevak, Rishbhak, Kakoli, Kshirkakoli, Mung, Urad, Jatamansi, Shatavari, Meda. This tea enhances sperm and balances the shukra dhatu in men.
- Anti-dermatitis Tea: Khadir, Haritaki, Amlaki, Haldi, Vidanga, Kaner, Amaltaas. This tea prevents skin inflammation and dermatitis.

Using Herbal Teas for Common Health Issues

Herbal teas are the soft yet powerful solution to all evils in life. Here's how you can solve everyday problems through these brews:

- Digestive problems: Feeling bloated or have indigestion? Try Digestive Tea with ginger, black pepper, and ajwain-it sets the digestive fire ablaze and removes toxins.
- Skin problem: If your skin loses its glow and suffers from rashes, manjistha, along with sandalwood, can be consumed as a Complexion Promoting Tea, which detoxifies and refills radiance.
- Fight Stress and Fatigue: Dates and raisins in Anti-Fatigue Tea work against fatigue and mental exhaustion. Nutrients and natural sugars revive energy levels.

- To Combat Allergies or Itching: Neem-Daruharidra Tonic Anti-Itching Tea combined with ½ tsp of Khadir and Arjun kills skin irritations and balances rakta and pitta dosha.
- To Lose or Gain Weight, Select the Weight-Reducing or Weight-Promoting Tea. Tea balances metabolism to needs, where dosha remains balanced.

Conclusion: One Sip of Wellness

Ayurveda's teas are remedies to heal and nourish. They can be ordinary drinks or specific remedies for certain health-related issues or things one needs daily to rejuvenate. These brews offer the simplest yet profound mode through which one can access the wisdom of Ayurveda for long-lasting vitality.

The more potent reason you are on your journey toward health and balance should be reminded by each sip-that there is harmony between nature and your body.

Chapter 20: The Power of One—Single Herbs

Single herbs are not just ingredients—they are powerful allies on the path to health and balance. Each herb possesses unique properties that can restore vitality, boost immunity, stimulate digestion, and cleanse the body. Restoring harmony between the doshas and the right herb at the right time makes them building blocks towards optimal health.

This chapter introduces 20 essential Ayurvedic herbs, detailing their medicinal properties and practical uses in daily life.

20 Must-Have Ayurvedic Herbs

Guduchi (Tinospora cordifolia)

- Medicinal Properties: Anti-inflammatory, adaptogenic, detoxifics, immunity booster.
- Uses: A powerful herb that strengthens the body against diseases and aids in detoxification. It is often used to treat joint pain, fever, and chronic fatigue.

Ashwagandha (Withania somnifera)

- Medicinal Properties: Adaptogenic, anti-stress, rejuvenating, anti-inflammatory.
- Uses: Known as *Indian Ginseng*, Ashwagandha fights stress, boosts energy, and improves sleep. It is excellent for Vata and Pitta balancing.

Manjistha (Rubia cordifolia)

- Medicinal Properties: Blood purifier, detoxifying, anti-inflammatory, skin healer.

- Uses: A well-known blood purifier that detoxifies the liver and kidneys. It is highly effective in treating acne, eczema, and skin rashes.

Haritaki (Terminalia chebula)

- Medicinal Properties: Laxative, digestive tonic, antioxidant, detoxifying.
- Uses: Promotes healthy digestion, supports bowel regularity, and benefits skin and eye health.

Amla (Phyllanthus emblica)

- Medicinal Properties: Rich in Vitamin C, antioxidant, immune-boosting, and anti-inflammatory.
- Uses: One of the most potent rejuvenating herbs in Ayurveda, Amla supports immune function, digestion, and anti-aging.

Bibhitaki (Terminalia bellirica)

- Medicinal Properties: Laxative, anti-inflammatory, antimicrobial, and rejuvenating.
- Uses: Helps detoxify the body, regulates bowel movements, and is beneficial for chronic cough, asthma, and respiratory issues.

Karanj (Pongamia pinnata)

- Medicinal Properties: Anti-inflammatory, antimicrobial, analgesic.
- Uses: Used to relieve arthritis pain, skin infections, and various inflammatory conditions.

Musta (Cyperus rotundus)

- Medicinal Properties: Digestive stimulant, anti-inflammatory, antispasmodic.
- Uses: A powerful digestive aid, Musta relieves bloating, gas, and menstrual discomfort.

Yastimadhu (Glycyrrhiza glabra)

- Medicinal Properties: Soothing, anti-inflammatory, expectorant, adaptogenic.
- Uses: Commonly known as *Licorice Root*, Yastimadhu helps with sore throats, coughs, ulcers, and hair health.

Bhringraj (Eclipta alba)

- Medicinal Properties: Liver tonic, hair growth promoter, anti-inflammatory.
- Uses: Known for detoxifying the liver and promoting healthy hair growth.

Jatamansi (Nardostachys jatamansi)

- Medicinal Properties: Sedative, anti-anxiety, neuroprotective, memory-enhancing.
- Uses: A deeply calming herb, Jatamansi is used to reduce stress and anxiety and enhance cognitive function.

Shankapushpi (Convolvulus pluricaulis)

- Medicinal Properties: Memory enhancer, anti-anxiety, sedative, cognitive support.
- Uses: Supports mental clarity and focus, and reduces anxiety.

Brahmi (Bacopa monnieri)

- Medicinal Properties: Cognitive enhancer, anti-anxiety, anti-inflammatory, adaptogenic.
- Uses: Improves memory, reduces stress, and benefits ADHD and cognitive function.

Gorakhmundi (Sphaeranthus indicus)

- Medicinal Properties: Antibacterial, anti-inflammatory, liver tonic.
- Uses: Supports liver function, boosts digestion, and promotes mental well-being.

Vacha (Acorus calamus)

- Medicinal Properties: Neuroprotective, anti-inflammatory, digestive stimulant.
- Uses: Known for enhancing speech fluency, cognitive function, and promoting gut health.

Usheer (Vetiveria zizanoides)

- Medicinal Properties: Cooling, calming, anti-inflammatory.
- Uses: A natural cooling herb, Usheer helps treat heat-related ailments, fever, and irritability.

Vasa (Adhatoda vasica)

- Medicinal Properties: Respiratory tonic, anti-cough, expectorant.
- Uses: Efficient for bronchitis, asthma, and chronic cough.

Anantmool (Hemidesmus indicus)

- Medicinal Properties: Detoxifying, anti-inflammatory, liver tonic.
- Uses: Cleanses toxins from the body, helps balance Pitta dosha, and supports liver function.

Pippali (Piper longum)

- Medicinal Properties: Digestive stimulant, expectorant, anti-inflammatory.
- Uses: Supports digestion and respiratory health, making it an excellent herb for Kapha-Vata balance.

Vidarikand (Pueraria tuberosa)

- Medicinal Properties: Tonic, anti-aging, strengthening.
- Uses: Helps boost stamina and strength and enhances reproductive health.

Integrating Herbs into Daily Life

Ayurvedic herbs are easy to incorporate into everyday routines:

- Teas & Decoctions: Brahmi tea enhances mental clarity, while Pippali tea supports digestion.
- Powders: Mixing Ashwagandha or Haritaki into warm water or smoothies boosts vitality.
- Oils & Topical Applications: Bhringraj and Vasa are used in hair and respiratory health formulations.

- Pastes: Manjistha and Guduchi can be applied externally for skin detoxification.

By integrating these herbs into your lifestyle, you can experience the profound healing power of Ayurveda.

A Story of Healing: Neha's Journey with Ayurvedic Herbs

Neha, a 28-year-old graphic designer, suffered from stress, fatigue, and digestive issues due to long working hours and an erratic lifestyle. A consultation with an Ayurvedic practitioner led her to try Ashwagandha for stress, Haritaki for digestion, and Brahmi for mental clarity.

She made simple changes to her daily routine—drinking Brahmi tea in the morning and taking Ashwagandha powder before bed. Neha felt a remarkable shift within weeks: her energy levels soared, digestion improved, and stress levels decreased. She restored her vitality and well-being by embracing the power of single Ayurvedic herbs.

Conclusion

Ayurvedic herbs offer robust natural solutions for maintaining health and balance. Whether you need mental clarity, anti-aging and liver tonics, or anti-inflammatory support, these 20 single herbs are a foundation for holistic well-being. By understanding and integrating them into your daily routine, you can harness the ancient wisdom of Ayurveda for lifelong vitality.

Chapter 21: Twenty-one Common Ailments and Herbs Used in Each Ailment

In each ailment, Ayurvedic practices offer a holistic approach to healing. Healing via herbs, essential for promoting wellness, is a prevalent aspect of Ayurveda. This chapter elucidates twenty-one common ailments and explores the corresponding herbs and formulations that address these conditions. It examines how these herbal remedies—when applied—restore balance and foster overall well-being. It is an exemplary account of the personal experiences of individuals undergoing Ayurvedic treatment, illustrating how such remedies can be integrated into daily health practices. However, the efficacy of these approaches can vary significantly because individual responses to treatment differ. Although many find success, it is essential to recognize the need for a tailored approach to each person's health needs.

Common Diseases Treated by Ayurveda

Ayurveda's healing system provides a comprehensive approach to health by addressing disease symptoms and underlying causes. Numerous common ailments are treated with Ayurvedic herbs; however, remarkable improvements two reported by patients are noteworthy. Although results vary, many individuals experience significant benefits because of this holistic method.

1. Arthritis

Numerous patients who have arthritis derive significant benefits from Ayurvedic medications. They often observe a reduction in joint swelling and diminished reliance on painkillers. Additionally, their ability to move freely increases. These medicinal remedies incorporate herbs such as Ginger and Ajmoda, which assist in preventing inflammatory conditions and alleviating pain. One herb with anti-inflammatory properties is Ashwagandha; this specific herb frequently mitigates flare-ups.

Herbs and formulations: Bala, Ginger, Turmeric, Ashwagandha, Mahayograj guggula, and Sinhanad guggula.

2. Crohn's Disease/Ulcerative Colitis

Patients experiencing inflammatory bowel disease (IBD) saw notable improvement. The inflammatory markers of calprotectin decreased significantly, and there were fewer signs of blood in the stool. Haritaki and Amla herbs are often utilized to treat and detoxify the digestive tract.

Herbs and Formulations: Haritaki, Amla, Guduchi, Dashmool, and Shankha Vati.

3. Hyperacidity/GERD/Acid Reflux

Ayurvedic treatment is beneficial for individuals suffering from hyperacidity and acid reflux. Herbal remedies that can reduce dependency on allopathic medications like antacids often yield prolonged relief. Licorice and Shankapushpi soothe the inner lining of the intestinal tract; amla effectively balances stomach acidity, thus contributing to overall wellness.

Herbs and Formulations: Licorice, Shankapushpi, Amla, Kamdudha, Avipattikar.

4. Hypertension

Ayurvedic herbs can remarkably reduce elevated blood pressure, especially when integrated into a broader lifestyle change that incorporates increased physical activity and alcohol avoidance. Arjuna and Ashwagandha are particularly effective; they possess the potential to fortify the heart, thus enabling it to regulate pressure more adeptly.

Herbs and Formulations: Arjuna, Ashwagandha, Sarpagandha, Gokshur.

5. Diabetes

Numerous individuals, many of whom seek alternative treatments, report a significant decline in blood sugar and A1c levels after commencing the use of Ayurvedic herbal supplements. Bitter Melon and Ginseng lower sugar levels and facilitate easier insulin absorption.

Herbs and Formulations: Bitter Melon, Ginseng, Fenugreek, Triphala, Haritaki, Chandraprabha vati.

6. Hair Fall

Bhringaraj and Amla are powerful herbs acknowledged for their capacity to stimulate hair growth; however, they also notably reduce hair loss. Many users observe that hair loss has decreased because of this, and hair has become thicker and healthier.

Herbs and Formulations: Bhringaraj, Amla, Yastimadhu, Jatamansi.

7. Hypothyroidism

Ayurvedic herbs such as Ashwagandha and Shatavari can effectively support proper thyroid functioning and hormonal balance. These herbs are often prescribed for enhancing thyroid function and boosting energy levels, which help diminish dependence on synthetic thyroid medications.

Herbs and Formulations: Ashwagandha, Shatavari, Yograj guggul, Chandraprabha vati.

8. Knee/Joint Pain

Turmeric and ginger are often used to alleviate knee and joint discomfort. These anti-inflammatory herbs significantly reduce inflammation levels, thus enhancing the range of motion; this, in turn, lessens pain intensity and promotes greater mobility. Herbs and Formulations: Turmeric, Ginger, Ajmodadi churn, Trayodashang guggul

9. Pain Muscular, Nerve

The Ayurvedic herbs Ashwagandha and Turmeric alleviate pain and inflammation associated with muscular or nerve pain in patients. Musta and boswellia also address conditions such as frozen shoulders and nerve pain.

Herbs and Formulations: Ashwagandha, Turmeric, Musta, Boswellia, mahayograj guggula, maharasnadi kashaya.

10. Skin Issues: Eczema, Psoriasis, Acne

Ayurvedic herbs such as Neem and Manjistha possess the potential to address myriad skin ailments: eczema, psoriasis, and acne. They purify the body, reducing inflammation, which is crucial for maintaining healthy skin. Furthermore, these herbs enhance blood flow, thus improving the appearance of bright, smooth skin.

Herbs and Formulations: Neem, Manjistha, Turmeric, Musta, Anantmool, Karanj, Khadir, Guduchi.

11. Sleep Disorders

Ayurveda is linked to enhanced sleep quality, insomnia, and tension alleviation. Brahmi and Jatamansi are commonly used herbs to soothe the nervous system and promote sleep quality.

Herbs and Formulations: Brahmi, Jatamansi, Shankapushpi, Ashwagandha

12. Tension Headache

Ayurvedic medicines have restrained the episodes and severity of stress headaches extensively. Brahmi and Shankapushpi are recognized for calming the brain and effectively alleviating stress; however, Lavender and Peppermint offer relief to the head and neck.

Herbs and Formulations: Brahmi, Shankapushpi, Lavender, Peppermint, Kamdudha, Sutshekhar.

13. Men's Health and Potency

In instances where an imbalance exists in rasa and shukra dhatus, male reproductive health may be adversely affected. Ayurvedic herbs that possess 'shukrakar' properties or shukra-producing enhance sperm quality; thus, they increase total semen volume per ejaculation. These herbs function as a tonic for men, aiming to elevate their overall vitality.

Herbs and Formulations: Kapikacchu, Safed musli, Ashwagandha, Vidarikand, Chandraprabha vati.

14. Alcohol and Opioid Addiction

Ayurvedic herbs are noted for their medicinal properties, which assist in alleviating withdrawal symptoms and cravings. Ashwagandha and Shankapushpi are particularly effective in reducing mood swings; however, Guduchi is crucial in supporting liver function and detoxifying the body.

Herbs and Formulations: Musta, Guduchi, Shankapushpi, Sariva, Patol, Kutki.

15. Autism/ADHD

Ayurveda enhances concentration and mitigates hyperactivity; Brahmi and Shankapushpi are especially effective in improving cognitive function. In contrast, Ashwagandha and Jatamansi are known to reduce restlessness and foster emotional balance.

Herbs and Formulations: Brahmi, Shankapushpi, Ashwagandha, Jatamansi

16. Women's Health (Hormonal Imbalance, Menstrual Health)

Shatavari and Ashwagandha are often administered regarding women's health to correct hormonal imbalances and menstrual issues. These herbs normalize menstrual cycles, boost fertility, and stabilize hormone levels.

Herbs and Formulations: Shatavari, Ashwagandha, Turmeric, Chandraprabha vati

17. Endometriosis

Ashoka and Turmeric are herbs recognized for reducing endometrial thickening. Thus, they relieve associated pain while promoting menstrual health and hormone regulation. Herbs and Formulations: Ashoka, Turmeric, Pushyanug.

18. Gastrointestinal issues (IBS, gas, bloating)

Ayurveda treats digestive disorders effectively with herbs like Triphala, Amla, and Ginger. These herbs balance Agni's digestive fire and cultivate healthy digestion, alleviating bloating, gas, and discomfort symptoms.

Herbs and Formulations: Triphala, Amla, Shunthi, Hingvastak churna, Sutshekhar.

19. Chronic Sinusitis

Chronic sinusitis, characterized by inflammation and swelling of the sinuses, usually leads to nasal congestion, headaches, and facial pain. According to Ayurveda, sinusitis is caused by an imbalance in Kapha dosha and the accumulation of Ama toxins. Some herbs like Pippali, Triphala, and Ginger help relieve sinusitis symptoms, purify the sinuses, diminish swelling, and support the respiratory system. Tulsi, or Holy Basil, is a well-known antimicrobial and anti-inflammatory agent.

Herbs and Formulations: Pippali, Triphala, Shunthi, Tulsi, Trikatu, Anu tail/Shadbindu tail (Nasya).

20. Chronic Fatigue Syndrome

Chronic Fatigue Syndrome (CFS) is characterized by prolonged fatigue that doesn't improve with rest. Ayurveda views CFS as a depletion of vital energy (Ojas). Ashwagandha, Shatavari, and Brahmi are herbs traditionally used to restore vitality, reduce fatigue, and rejuvenate the body and mind. These adaptogenic herbs help the body better manage stress, improve stamina, and support the nervous system.

Herbs and Formulations: Ashwagandha, Shatavari, Brahmi, Yastimadhu, Vidarikand, Bala.

21. Tics

Involuntary muscular movements, sometimes known as tics, can feel disorganized. Ashwagandha and Brahmi are recognized as helpful in reducing nervous system excitability. These herbs relax the mind and minimize tic episodes.

Herbs and Formulations: Ashwagandha, Brahmi, Gorakhmundi, Shankapushpi, Brahmi, Vacha.

Practical Application in Everyday Health

Incorporating Ayurvedic herbs into one's daily regimen can significantly enhance overall health and well-being; however, several straightforward methods exist to integrate these natural remedies into life: for instance, consider herbal teas such as those made with brahmi, turmeric, or ashwagandha, which can provide soothing, digestive, or stress-relieving benefits. Furthermore, topical applications of herbal oils—like neem oil for acne or Bhringraj oil for scalp and hair health—can effectively alleviate skin discomfort and irritation. Mixing Triphala powder with warm water can aid digestion, but taking ashwagandha powder may help improve energy levels and reduce stress. You might also consider daily supplements, such as adding amla powder to smoothies or consuming turmeric capsules as a regular anti-inflammatory measure. Integrating these herbs into lifestyle can address fundamental health concerns while promoting longevity and balance. However, Ayurveda advocates for healing by restoring harmony among body, mind, and spirit naturally and holistically.

Chapter 22: The Detoxifying and Rejuvenating Force – Panchakarma Therapies

Panchakarma Therapies of Ayurveda are evident in detoxification and rejuvenation to keep the body, mind, and spirit healthy. The foundation for this ancient science is Panchakarma- a group of five therapeutic detoxification techniques geared towards removing Aama or toxins from the system, restoring the doshic balance, and helping the body regain proper functioning. These detoxifying and rejuvenating therapies are inherent to Ayurvedic health care. This chapter focuses on the most critical detoxifying Panchakarma therapies, which include Vaman, Virechan, Basti, Nasya, and Leech Therapy. Nasya Therapy is also a detoxifying and rejuvenating treatment that falls under this category, although only Nasya will be elaborated upon in the following chapter. The next chapter describes Shirodhara, which is also classified as one of the rejuvenating therapies. Since the height of mental health issues has reached today's world, Shirodhara and Nasya have received relatively more attention.

Lisa, 38, a professional, suffered from chronic fatigue, severe allergies, and persistent brain fog after years of work in stressful information technology industry environments. She learned most treatments stopped the symptoms from occurring, which left her far more tired and disconnected. Panchakarma opened doors for her when a friend proposed that she do Ayurveda. Her first detoxification in Vaman kicked out years' worth of toxins caused by Kapha, letting her sinus clear and allergies minimized. The easing of her digestion started with Pitta balancing done by Virechan, enabling her to obtain more energy. Lastly, she was given Basti therapy, which used herbal oils to soothe the agitated Vata within her while resolving the stiffness in joints she had suffered for years from such a sedentary lifestyle. She was given Nasya therapy, which cleared out her nasal passage and cleared up her thoughts. Leech therapy healed inflammation in her skin and energized her. The whole range of treatments cleaned up her body and turned her to health and peace; it was, however, no cakewalk.

Realizing the impact of her lifestyle on her mind, Lisa welcomed Shirodhara therapy in the subsequent sessions to relieve stress and achieve emotional balance. At the end of her Panchakarma journey, she felt rejuvenated and gained valuable insights into maintaining balance in her everyday life. However, she realized that it was a process that had to be achieved daily because it required constant effort. She was grateful for such an experience, but it was far from the end.

Detox Techniques-Panchakarma

It denotes "five actions" or "five therapies"; five methods to eliminate deep-set impurities. They are vastly diverse from person to person. Prakriti is one's body constitution, dosha imbalance, or special conditions at the level of being. They help a person detoxify his body, improve digestion, and correct imbalance, thus achieving body, mind, and spiritual harmony. Before Panchakarma, there lies a preparatory phase known as Purva Karma. This includes internal and external oleation called Snehana and fomentation Swedana to loosen and prepare the body to evacuate the toxins. Paschat Karma means post-treatment care, done after significant therapies, to help the body recover with a positive approach toward revivification. Vaman, Virechan, Basti, Nasya, and Leech Therapy—benefits.

1. Vaman or Therapeutic Emesis

Vaman therapy, a technique of oral medication, evokes therapeutic vomiting, which expels toxins from the mouth. It is helpful in cases of aggravated Kapha dosha, asthma, bronchitis, and chronic sinusitis. Sage Charak beautifully depicts Vaman as "Just like the crops die out when the water supply is blocked; diseases dry out when all toxins are evacuated from the body by Vaman." But then again, the treatment is highly potent, and therefore, it should not be given unless a patient is fully healthy enough to endure the aftermath. The treatments can be too effective, so they are only used carefully and under various circumstances.

It removes excess mucus from the respiratory tract. It regulates Kapha dosha and aids digestion. It also helps overcome skin disorders like acne and eczema caused by toxin accumulation. It relieves allergy symptoms and respiratory disorders by reducing the feeling of heaviness, numbness, stiffness, drowsiness, and lethargy. Though these benefits are great, the remedy must be consumed wisely.

Weight management technique

To make the patient vomit, herbal medicines, such as madanphal and kashaya with honey and salt, are given to him. He is hydrated and kept resting to regain balance. This process becomes uncomfortable. Patients do not like it; they are frightened by the side effects. But he is still in recovery.

2. Virechan or Therapeutic Purgation

Virechan purifies the body by causing continuous bowel movements to remove toxins from the gut. It is used in Pitta disorders, such as skin infections, digestive issues, or increased heat. While Raman evacuates undigested doshas mainly from the stomach, Virechan evacuates toxic doshas already digested and present in the intestines. Therefore, depending on individual conditions, Raman can be finished faster than Virechan.

Benefits:

- It cleanses the liver and gallbladder.

It alleviates hyperacidity and chronic skin problems, such as psoriasis, eczema, and dermatitis, but might work differently on others. Since it gives instant relief, there may not be a total cure. So, one should consider visiting a physician before this medicine alone for their problem.

- Eases chronic constipation.

Balances Pitta dosha one and reduces inflammation, improving the body's general metabolic function. However, this must be done concerning the holistic approach to health, as many factors are involved in wellness. Even though some might not consider these associations, they are significant in balancing.

- Diabetes and herpes.

Mild laxatives or herbal preparations – like abhayadi modak, castor oil, Triphala, and trivrit lehyam – flush the colon, ensuring it is thoroughly cleansed. If the vire chan does not come following herbal preparations, then a mildly hot bag fomentation on the stomach area should be resorted to. If the bowel movement is scanty, take khichdi at night and repeat vire chan the next day; however, that may not always be necessary as results can vary. Though effective, some may find it less palatable than they had anticipated.

3. Basti or Medicated Enema

Basti treatment involves administering medicated oils or herbal decoctions through the rectum to purify and nourish the body. It is one of the most potent treatments in Ayurveda, especially for Vata disorders. Though effective, people may be apprehensive about the process, which requires a certain degree of openness and trust. However, the benefits can be colossal and contribute to overall well-being.

Benefits :

It kills chronic constipation and bloating, crucial for preventing Irritable Bowel Syndrome. It also decreases the level of Vata dosha; however, it balances nervous disorders and reduces sleep disorders. Due to its anti-inflammatory properties, it helps maintain joint health by decreasing inflammation and stiffness. It increases reproductive health and improves immunity, but the mechanism is very complex.

- It helps in curing kidney stones and gallstones.
- Reduces inflammation in the colon.
- Uttar basti evacuates toxins from the uterus.

Procedure: Oil-based Anuvasana or herbal decoction-based Niruha enemas are administered according to the patient's condition; however, the treatment is rejuvenating and nourishing for the colon. Uttar Basti is an oil enema administered to women through vaginal passage, though its application may vary. This treatment is effective because it addresses specific health needs.

4. Nasya or Nasal Therapy

The administration of medicated oils or herbal liquids through the nasal passages detoxifies and strengthens the head and neck region, which is very beneficial for both Kapha and Vata imbalances. However, one needs to keep in mind the variability in effects. Though the practice is generally considered positive, it must be attended to with caution because responses can vary enormously from one person to another.

Benefits:

It clears sinus congestion and allergies and tones the breath. It also strengthens the faculties of mind, thought clarity, and mental pacification. Mainly, it helps against epilepsy. Headaches, migraines, and sleep disorders are reduced; however, it also sharpens the smoothness, stability, and depth of the voice, purifying the sense organs. Besides, this medicine strengthens the joints and muscles of the face and scalp. The process involves the following: after a preparatory massage and steam, the herbal oil or liquid is gradually introduced into the nostrils with gentle massage and rest. Anu tail is one of the most widely used oils for nasya. It contains pitta-balancing herbs, such as Chandan, Bala, cardamom, usher, cinnamon, musta, and anantmool. Other oils used for nasya are shadbindu tail and panchendriyavardhan tail.

5. Leech Therapy or Jalouka Therapy

Many of the benefits that leech therapy, one of the traditional methods of medical practice that purify the blood, gives are as follows: First and foremost, medicinal leeches that draw impure blood are fresh-water ones. Therefore, they speed up blood flow and reduce body inflammation. Sage Vagbhatta metaphorically states that the leech can differentiate between pure blood and one that contains toxins, just like the 'swan draws milk from a mixture of water and milk.' But this is interesting because it points out the natural abilities of these creatures, although some may wonder whether it works.

Benefits:

It eliminates skin diseases like acne, rosacea, psoriasis, and eczema. It also reduces inflammation intensity, and the degree of pain caused in joints and arthritis is minimized. In addition, it promotes blood flow alongside the cleaning of blood. It heals chronic wounds and varicose veins. Process: Medicinal leeches are applied to specific areas of the body. After they fall off themselves, the wound is cleaned, and the patient is advised to rest and rehydrate. The leech is cleaned by submerging it in turmeric water. This treatment has some potential since some patients do great with it. It may sound rather unorthodox to some, but it works for many.

Preparation and Aftercare

Preparation or Purva Karma

Pre-treatment is also crucial to the success of Panchakarma; this involves Snehana or oleation, where medicated oils are used internally and externally to make the body soft, relax, and render it supple. Swedana: Fomentation or herbal steam is given to open up pores. It lets toxins leave the body system. Dietary adaptation is essential; it must be a light, easy-to-digest diet to prepare the digestive system for detoxification. However, one has to be careful since each person's requirements may differ, which can go a long way in determining the effectiveness of the treatment.

Aftercare Panchakarma or Paschat Karma

Recovery is the final stage of Panchakarma, which guarantees a smooth healing process for the body. This stage encompasses various elements.

- Dietary guidelines state that one should progressively consume lighter to heavier foods, starting with light, warm food. For example, rice water kanji on day 1, mung dal soup on day 2, and khichdi on day 3 are suggested.

- Herbal Support is also essential; continuous intake of herbal teas and preparations helps revive.
- Lifestyle Changes include yoga, meditation, and conscious living that maintain balance and health. Incorporating these is quite important.

Finally, incorporating Panchakarma into a healthy lifestyle is not detoxification; instead, it is a fantastic healing and rejuvenation process in which imbalances are tackled in their roots. All the toxin removals can be done through these therapies, which treat entirely the body, mind, and soul to look healthy. While it may include the detoxifying property of Vaman and Virechan, the nourishing effect of Basti, or even the targeted healing by Nasya and Leech Therapy, Panchakarma is that journey that leads one toward re-establishing harmony and radiating life. The method stands the test of time for anyone seeking deep detoxification and rejuvenation—Panchakarma is an intense Ayurvedic healing process. Still, it is crucial to remember that the process will vary from individual to individual due to different needs.

Conclusion: Adopting Panchakarma for Healthy Living

Panchakarma therapies are not detoxification alone but a deep healing and rejuvenation process. By dealing with the root causes of imbalances and removing toxins from the body, these therapies give a healthy body, mind, and soul an all-around way of healing. Whether it is the cleansing power of Vaman and Virechan, the nourishing effects of Basti, or the targeted healing of Nasya and Leech Therapy, Panchakarma provides a transformative experience that restores harmony and vitality. For anyone seeking deep detoxification and rejuvenation, Panchakarma is a powerful Ayurvedic approach to healing that stands the test of time.

Chapter 23: The Tranquil Mind – Shirodhara Therapy

Healing is not limited to diet or herbs in Ayurveda. Treatments rejuvenate the body, mind, and spirit. In the previous chapter, we discussed the five detoxification therapies. Other therapies, such as Shirodhara, treat specific imbalances, reduce stress, improve digestion, and enhance overall well-being. This chapter explains Shirodhara, a treatment known for calming the mind and enhancing mental clarity, thus improving health and well-being.

Shirodhara: An Overview

This is one of the traditional treatments practiced under Ayurveda therapy wherein there is constant, rhythmic dripping of warm medicated oil or other liquid medicines onto the forehead and third eye (the region between the eyebrows). This name comes from the two Sanskrit roots: the term for the word "Shirodhara" is broken into 'Shiro,' head, and 'Dhara' – flow or stream. This technique, more than three thousand years old, involves deep relaxation in mental clarity and feeling inner peace. It is sometimes called "liquid meditation" since it allows people to settle into a peaceful, meditative mindset.

According to Ayurveda, Shirodhara balances the Vata and Pitta doshas, which govern the nervous system and mind. The steady flow of warm oil on the third eye soothes the central nervous system, balances the mind, frees stored-up stress, and achieves emotional balance. It is one of the most in-demand treatments for stress, anxiety, and sleep disorders and is available in Ayurvedic wellness centers.

Benefits to the mind

The therapeutic result of Shirodhara is deep and wide, bringing about some benefits for a person's physical and mental well-being. Some such benefits include:

- Relief from Anxiety and Stress: Shirodhara's initial benefit is stress and anxiety relief. The gentle, rhythmic flow of warm oil down the forehead stimulates the parasympathetic nervous system, relaxing the body and inducing a state of serenity. This kind of stress relief has immediate and long-term effects on mental and physical health.
- Mental Clarity and Focus: Shirodhara has a balancing effect on the mind. This therapy improves mental miasma or mental fogginess, resulting in clarity and focus. The calming of the nervous system removes distractions and worries; the person starts feeling fresh and clear-minded. This is the reason it can be considered an excellent treatment for people suffering from mental fatigue or a lack of focus. The deep relaxation offered by Shirodhara soothes excessive thoughts causing anxiety. It has been found to have a therapeutic effect on the Vata dosha, which causes anxiety, worry, and fear. Thus, daily sessions reduce stress and attune the mind to an emotional balance.
- Improved Sleep: Shirodhara is perfect for people with insomnia or insomnia. It relaxes the mind and controls the nervous system, giving more refreshing and profound sleep.

The effect of Shirodhara reduces the impact by letting the individual sleep early and during the night with sound, long-lasting sleep.

- Emotional Balance: Shirodhara is sometimes referred to as an emotional reboot. It frees pent-up emotions and deep-seated stress, thus providing emotional healing and balance. This is useful for trauma, depression, or overpowering emotions, as it imparts a feeling of inner peace and stability.
- Hypertension: Shirodhara has emerged as a favorable treatment for patients suffering from hypertension. It helps calm the nervous system, removing stress, which is one of the main reasons for high blood pressure. During the therapy, the parasympathetic response is triggered, creating relaxation and lowering cortisol levels; hence, blood pressure is appropriately balanced. Continued treatments enhance the emotional state of being and also give relief at a physical level, making them holistic in managing hypertension.

The Procedure and Therapeutic Effect

This therapy, called Shirodhara, is a very relaxing, meditative experience. Several carefully coordinated steps contribute to the calming and therapeutic effect of the procedure. The steps followed are as follows:

- Preparing:

Before the Shirodhara treatment, a short Abhyanga is usually performed to relax the muscles and prepare the body for the treatment. This helps open up the channels of circulation so that the oils applied in Shirodhara are adequately absorbed.

- Setting:

The treatment is usually administered in a peaceful, quiet ambiance, sometimes with soothing background music and dim lighting that helps to increase relaxation even further. The patient will be asked to lie on a comfortable massage table, typically supporting their head with a small pillow or cushion. Ayurvedic oils or herbal liquids are chosen based on the person's dosha and the individual requirement. Shirodhara's oils are sesame, bhringraj, or medicated oils infused with herbs like Brahmi, sandalwood, and licorice. These oils are selected according to the patient's mental state and dosha imbalances.

- Oil Pouring:

The central part of the therapy involves continuously pouring warm oil over the forehead in a steady stream, moving from one side of the forehead to the other. The oil flows gently over the third eye (the space between the eyebrows), which is believed to stimulate the Ajna chakra, the center of intuition, mental clarity, and consciousness. This process typically lasts 30-45 minutes.

- Post-Treatment Rest:

After the oil has been applied, the patient is rested for a few minutes to allow the full penetrative effect of the oil to reach the skin. Throughout these minutes, stress in the body continues to reduce, and the mind feels calm and serene. Some therapists provide minimal cranial massage to increase the depth of relaxation.

- Final Cleaning:

Scalp treatment usually ends with mild rubbing to remove all existing tenses. After this, the doctor carefully wipes the redundant oil and tells the patient to drink as much warm water or herbal tea as possible to speed up the detox process.

Conclusion: A Soothing Mind

Shirodhara therapy is a healing process by which the mind and body are healed. It deeply relaxes the nervous system, clears mental fog, reduces anxiety, and improves sleep. Shirodhara is one of the most powerful Ayurvedic tools for fostering mental clarity, emotional balance, and deep inner peace, whether used for rejuvenation or as a regular wellness routine for people seeking maximum benefit.

Shirodhara is a haven for peace for anyone looking to step away from stress and find long-term wellness. Let its healing energy work magic, and discover its profound impact on your mind, body, and spirit.

Chapter 24: Nasya – The Breath of Purity and Ear Oil Therapy (Karna Puran)

Having in-depth knowledge about the physiological and psychological relationship of the human body, Ayurveda gives particular importance to purifying and nourishing sensory organs for complete well-being and balance. Nasya and Karna Puran, or ear oil treatment, is one of the healing processes for sound breath, clear-mindedness, and balancing of the sense organs: detoxifying and rejuvenating the nasal channel and ears allows for deep well-being.

Nasya: The Process and Benefits

Nasya is an Ayurvedic treatment in which medicated oils or herbal liquids are dropped into the nasal cavity. It is one of the five procedures of Panchakarma, and the therapy is very effective in treating head, neck, and respiratory disorders. The nose is a gateway to the head and, therefore, a portal through which this de-toxifying and enriching therapy enters the head.

Procedure

- Preparation: This is the initial treatment, during which facial muscles are relaxed and nasal channels are opened using mild massage with warm oil.
- Steam Fomentation: Herbal steam is applied over the face and neck to loosen the toxins inside and open the pores on the face.

- Application of Oil: Mild application of warm medicated oil like Anu Taila or Shadbindu Taila, drop by drop, through both nostrils. The patient is asked to breathe inward so that they can enable oil to enter sinus cavities.
- Post-treatment Care: After the oil is applied, the forehead and neck region are lightly massaged, and the patient rests.

Benefits

- Respiratory Health: Nasya removes excess mucus, reduces nasal congestion, and increases smooth breathing. This treatment is beneficial for cases with sinusitis, allergies, and asthma.
- Mental Clarity: The treatment revs up the brain and calms down the nervous system, thus making one more alert, focused, and concentrated.
- Headache: Repeated Nasya will help prevent headaches, migraines, and head and neck tension.
- Skin Condition: Detoxification in the scalp area allows for healthy and bright skin.
- Sleep: The soothed mind will allow better management of insomnia and disturbed sleep cycles.

Respiratory and Mental Well-being Improvement

Ravi (45) is a middle-school teacher with persistent sinus congestion and chronic fatigue that worsens every season. His days are laborious, marked by labored breathing, frequent colds, and exhaustion that persists even after resting. As time passes, the pressure from these issues starts to take a toll on his energy and health.

He went for a Nasya treatment. Under the guidance of an Ayurvedic doctor, he started a course that gradually detoxified his nose and sinuses. During this process, debris began to clear up the nasal cavity and sinuses, and he started witnessing a significant improvement in breathing. He felt stronger for extended periods since his stamina had increased, and he wasn't tired throughout the day.

The benefits were not just physical. Ravi had also been suffering from mental fogginess and stress due to overwork for many years. Nasya proved to be a boon to his nervous system. As it helped in balancing his Vata dosha, Ravi felt his anxiety reduce, his focus improve, and his emotional well-being grow. By the end of his therapy, Ravi felt healthy, more centered, and ready to face life with renewed vitality.

Ear Oil Therapy (Karna Puran): A Panacea for All Afflictions

Karna Puran, or ear oil therapy, is another crucial Ayurvedic treatment that nourishes and protects the ears. In Ayurveda, the ears are considered a vital sensory organ; proper care is essential to maintaining balance in the body and mind.

Procedure

- Preparation: The massage commences with warm oil surrounding the ears, neck, and head to induce relaxation.

- Application of Oil: Medicated oil, usually Bala Taila or Dashamoola Taila, is warmed to a comfortable temperature. The patient is positioned on one side, and the oil is carefully dripped into the ears.
- Resting Phase: The patient is maintained in this position for some minutes to allow the penetration of the oil that fills and lubricates the ear canal.
- Drainage and Cleaning: After the drainage, the oil is let out, and a soft cloth cleans the ear

Benefits

- Improving Hearing: Karna Puran improves hearing by flushing out the obstacles and feeding the ear nerves.
- Tinnitus Relief: It reduces ringing or buzzing in the ears, effectively brought on by Vata's overactivity.
- Reduces Stress: Therapy relaxes the nervous system and calms anxiety, insomnia, and restlessness.
- Supports Equilibrium and Coordination: Maintaining ear health aids the inner ear in equilibrium and spatial orientation.
- Provides Relief in Pain: It reduces infections or environmental causes of earaches and inflammation.

Conclusion: Breathing and Listening to Wellness

Nasya and Karna Puran are not just therapies—they are rituals of self-care that rejuvenate the senses, enhance respiratory and auditory health, and restore mental clarity. In a world filled with noise and stress, these Ayurvedic treatments offer a sanctuary of calm, helping individuals reconnect with their inner harmony. Nasya purifies breathing, and Karna Puran offers soothing endearment. Such therapies remind us of the immense interconnection between our sensory organs and general well-being. If done regularly, these practices will pave the way toward a balanced life of vibrancy and serenity.

Chapter 25: Herbal Allies – Prominent Herbs in Panchakarma

Panchakarma is an Ayurvedic detoxification and rejuvenation of the body in general. Whether the treatment will go well depends on the therapeutic uses of many herbs. They play a massive role in purifying the body, generating tissues, and restoring doshas to balance. This chapter examines key herbs employed in Panchakarma therapy, elucidating their healing attributes and significance in detoxification. Although the advantages are considerable, one must consider individual reactions of the body because not all herbs will produce the same outcomes for every individual.

Main Herbs Used in Panchakarma Therapy

1. Herbs Used in Vaman

The Vaman treatment completely removes excess Kapha dosha, which can cause many health issues and throw out mucus and toxins from the stomach. However, this process is arduous and requires proper preparation and guidance. Although many individuals may encounter considerable relief, others may find it somewhat uncomfortable. Because of this, it is crucial to approach the treatment with care and comprehension.

- Madanphal (*Randia dumetorum*)

Healing Properties: Madhanphal exhibits emetic actions (which are regulated), alleviates excess Kapha, and desiccates surplus mucus.

Applications: It mitigates respiratory congestion, asthma, and conditions related to skin (caused by an overabundance of Kapha).

- Yastimadhu (*Glycyrrhiza glabra*)

Healing Properties: Yastimadhu has anti-inflammatory effects (which relieve the digestive tract) and a balancing influence on Pitta.

Applications: It decreases acidity and calms the throat and stomach lining during Vaman therapy.

- Kutaj (*Holarrhena antidysenterica*)

Healing Properties: Kutaj's properties encompass astringent, antibacterial, and anti-diarrheal effects.

Applications: Enhances digestive health and mitigates gastrointestinal inflammation before Vaman.

- Pippali (*Piper longum*)

Healing Properties: The properties of Pippali are its carminative effects (which stimulate Agni — the digestive fire) and mobilize toxins within the body.

Applications: It assists in eliminating excess Kapha, alleviates respiratory blockages, and enhances lung function.

2. Herbs Used in Virechan

Virechan therapy (recognized for its detoxifying attributes) purifies the liver, intestines, and gallbladder; thus, it effectively diminishes excess Pitta dosha. However, this procedure necessitates careful contemplation because it can influence other bodily functions. Although it is advantageous, one must proceed with caution.

- Munakka (*Vitis vinifera*)

Healing Properties: Munakka exhibits

(a) relatively gentle purgative action and

(b) a cooling, nourishing effect on the body.

Applications: It helps alleviate bowel movements by mitigating inflammation in the intestine.

- Vacha (*Acorus calamus*)

Healing Properties: Vacha functions as a stimulant, carminative, and decongestant.

Applications: It effectively removes toxins, eliminates blockages in arteries, improves speech, and cleanses the gastrointestinal tract.

- Amaltas (*Cassia fistula*)

Healing Properties: Amaltas is a mild purgative, exhibits anti-inflammatory attributes, and imparts a cooling effect.

Applications: This particular herb targets the intestines, especially concerning ailments linked to bowel and liver conditions.

- Triphala

Healing Properties: Triphala balances three doshas, promotes good digestion, and eliminates toxins from the gut.

Applications: Triphala is the foundation for Virechan. It cleanses the intestinal system, aiding in establishing a regular stool routine.

3. Herbs Used in Basti

Basti operates at the apex of Vata Dosha and efficiently eliminates toxins from all bodily systems, enhancing tissue nutrition.

- Sariva (*Hemidesmus Indicus*)

Healing Properties: Sariva purifies the blood and has an anti-inflammatory cooling effect.

Applications: Its usage is multifaceted, as it nourishes kidneys and effectively removes toxins. However, it also calms doshas, particularly Vata and Pitta, which are necessary for maintaining balance.

- Gokhshura (*Tribulus Terrestris*)

Healing Properties: Gokshura's properties, including diuretic effects, are noteworthy; they also demonstrate anti-inflammatory traits and aid in rejuvenation.

Applications: It addresses urinary disorders and improves sexual health, consequently offering vital support to the colon.

- Erand (*Ricinus communis*)

Healing Properties: Erand's properties encompass lubricating, purgative, and anti-inflammatory effects.

Applications: Often involves basti, where castor oil is utilized. This method is particularly effective as it alleviates symptoms of constipation and Vata imbalance pain in joints.

- Punarnava (*Boerhavia diffusa*)

Healing Properties: The properties of Punarnava involve diuretic, anti-edematous, and detoxifying effects.

Applications: It alleviates symptoms of water retention, which can be very uncomfortable, nourishes the liver, and rekindles the colon.

- Guduchi (*Tinospora cordifolia*)

Healing Properties: Guduchi is an immunity booster, anti-inflammatory, and rejuvenating.

Applications: Nourishes tissues, enhances immunity, and supports detoxification post-Basti therapy.

4. Herbs Used in Nasya

Nasya detoxifies an individual's head, neck, and respiratory channels and balances the Vata and Kapha doshas. However, this process is not mechanical because it entails a more profound connection to well-being. Although the outcomes may differ from person to person, the significance of sustaining this balance cannot be overstated.

- Chandan (*Santalum album*)

Healing Properties: Chandan exhibits cooling, anti-inflammatory, and anti-pitta effects.

Applications: It clears nasal passages and mitigates Pitta while simultaneously soothing the lungs.

- Bala (*Sida cordifolia*)

Healing Properties: Bala's healing properties include its function as a nerve tonic, strengthener, and reviver. Applications: Nurturing the nerves can enhance mental cognition and clear the nostrils.

- Musta (*Cyperus rotundus*)

Healing Properties: Musta's properties encompass its function as a detoxifying agent, anti-inflammatory effects, and laxative qualities.

Applications: Clearing the head, balancing Kapha, and sharpening mental clarity.

5. Herbs Used in Leech Therapy

Leech therapy aims to purify the blood of impurities, diminish inflammation, and improve circulation. However, it is crucial to recognize that this technique has encountered skepticism from various medical professionals. Although numerous anecdotal reports exist regarding its efficacy, scientific data remains inconclusive. This uncertainty raises questions surrounding its broader application. Because of these considerations, those contemplating leech therapy should advance cautiously but will quickly discover it to be advantageous in specific situations.

- Turmeric (*Curcuma longa*)

Healing properties: Turmeric has noteworthy healing properties, including anti-inflammatory, antiseptic, and blood-purifying effects.

Applications: particularly significant in diminishing inflammation and swelling. This, in turn, accelerates the healing process and can mitigate the risk of infections.

6. Herbs Used in Shirodhara

Shirodhara employs a combination of soothing and invigorating herbs that synchronize the mind while reducing stress within the nervous system.

- Brahmi (*Bacopa monnieri*)

Healing Properties: Brahmi enhances mental capacity, reduces stress, and improves memory.

Applications: Shirodhara oils, known for their soothing qualities, pacify the mind and alleviate anxiety from the body; however, they also function as sleep inducers.

- Ashwagandha (*Withania somnifera*)

Healing Properties: The healing properties of Ashwagandha are noteworthy; it alleviates stress and refreshes the mind.

Applications: When the nervous system is engaged and fortified, Ashwagandha reduces fatigue and improves emotional equilibrium.

- Jatamansi (*Nardostachys jatamansi*)

Healing Properties: Jatamansi's properties are soothing, sedative, and grounding.

Applications: It controls mental unrest, cures insomnia, and calms the nervous system.

Healing Properties and Usage

The previously mentioned herbs are utilized independently and in combination to produce oils, pastes, and decoctions that enhance their effectiveness. For example,

- Medicated Oils:

Ashwagandha, Neem, and Brahmi are combined with sesame or coconut oils for treatments such as Shirodhara, Abhyanga, and Karna Puran, which deliver calming benefits and nurture the mind and body.

- Herbal Decoctions:

Triphala, Guduchi, and Turmeric are mainly administered when patients undergo Virechan and Basti treatments because both processes facilitate detoxification and dosha balancing.

- Nasya Oils:

Preparing for Nasya treatment may include medicated oils, such as Pippali and Brahmi, to preserve the mind's and lungs' health. However, it is essential to recognize that the efficacy of these treatments can vary significantly based on individual circumstances.

Awareness of the Detoxification Process

The detoxification process inherent in Panchakarma fundamentally depends on using various herbs. For example,

- Mobilization:

A range of herbs, such as Neem and Triphala, dismantle numerous internal toxins within the body, passing them to the gut for excretion.

- Elimination:

Vaman, Virechan, and Basti therapies use herbs like Pippali and Guggul to eliminate toxins from the body.

- Rejuvenation:

Once detoxification has been established, incorporating herbs like Shatavari and Ashwagandha help to rebuild strength, revitalize tissues, and restore strength with vigor. This herbal combination ensures that the Panchakarma treatment is effective.

Conclusion: The Power of Herbal Allies

Panchakarma functions synergistically to attain the highest effectiveness in detoxification and rejuvenation. Each herb demonstrates a unique mechanism of action that enhances its intrinsic properties; thus, it fosters dosha balance, ultimately resulting in overall wellness and vitality. The purifying attributes of Triphala, the invigorating effects of Ashwagandha, and the soothing influence of Brahmi are all realized in Panchakarma therapies that employ these medicinal herbs. In this context, Ayurveda offers a pathway as timeless as history—guiding practitioners toward a thorough restoration of health and energy. However, this harmonious methodology emphasizes the significance of merging traditional wisdom with contemporary practices because, although change is inevitable, the essence of these ancient practices remains vital.

Chapter 26: Yoga and Ayurveda- A Harmonious Union

Yogic and Ayurvedic knowledge of ancient Indian sciences were closely entwined in sister disciplines. Ayurveda aims to heal human beings holistically, including all the functions of the body and the mind. In turn, yoga is intended to maintain such balance through specific disciplines such as bodily postures, breathing control, and meditation. This composite discipline offers a way toward health encompassing physical, mental, and spiritual dimensions of well-being.

Yoga in Ayurveda is not a set of exercises but a necessity for balancing doshas, enhancing Agni, and eliminating accumulated Ama. By assimilating with the philosophy of Ayurveda, Yoga ensures that the body is a stable enough vessel to hold the mind to bring peace and balance to life.

The Relation of Yoga to Ayurveda

Ayurveda and Yoga share a common objective: the body, mind, and spirit must harmonize with the rhythm of nature. Ayurveda further states that an individual's doshas, Vata, Pitta, and Kapha, work best when balanced. Yoga offers such equilibrium through a stable body, a sharp mind, and an emotionally resistant personality.

Different yoga practices are to be given depending upon the Prakriti of a person and the imbalances in doshas.

- Vata Disorder: Calming, grounding postures with slow movement and deep breathing to balance the nervous system.
- Pitta Disorder: Cooling, restorative postures, and practices to calm irritability and overheating.
- Kapha Disorder: Dynamic yoga flows stimulate the body to reduce the lack of movement.

Ayurveda establishes the conceptual basis for an individual's requirements, while Yoga provides one with the skills to fulfill those requirements.

Pranayama and Yoga Practices for Health

The science of breath regulation in yoga is identical to the concepts of Ayurveda. Several pranayama forms have varied effects on doshas, which help cleanse, calm the mind, and rejuvenate the body.

- Anulom Vilom (Alternate Nostril Breathing)

Ayurvedic View: It balances the Vata and central nervous system (sympathetic and parasympathetic).

Benefits: Purifies and harmonizes the flow of Prana through the energy channels, calming agitated thoughts and removing tension.

- Bhastrika (Bellows Breath)

Ayurvedic View: It stimulates body energy, sets Agni, and balances Kapha.

Benefits: Increases oxygenation, clears lung condition, and boosts mental energy.

- Kapal Bhati (Skull-Shining Breath)

Ayurvedic View: It cleanses toxins, helps in digestion, and helps reduce Kapha-induced heaviness, especially in visceral organs.

Benefits: Elevates concentration and improves digestion to support extra fat burn-off.

- Sheetali (Cooling Breath)

Ayurveda View: Smoothen the pitta as it cools the body and gives a scorching feeling.

Benefits: Relieves the imbalance from excess heat and relaxes the mind.

- Ujjayi (Controlled Breathing)

Ayurveda View - Synchronize your brain by controlling the Vata and Pitta.

Benefits: It balances thyroid hormones, strengthens the lungs, and enhances concentration.

Thus, Pranayama and Ayurveda can be powerful tools for balancing and resisting various diseases. Together, they can also build mental and physical strength.

Teaching Yoga in an Ayurvedic Setting

In an Ayurvedic lifestyle, yoga starts by learning about your body's needs. Ayurveda emphasizes Dinacharya or daily routine, and practicing yoga and pranayama are integral to maintaining dosha balance. A typical Ayurvedic lifestyle morning might be something like this:

- Abhyanga, or self-oil massage, to prepare the body for movement.
- Pranayama awakens the respiratory system, lowers cortisol levels, and rejuvenates the prana.
- Yoga Asanas, tailored to your dosha, invigorate and align the body.

For Example:

Gentle asanas, such as Child's Pose or Seated Forward Fold, can help a Vata-prone person balance his uncontrolled movements.

Cooling postures such as Moon Salutations or Reclining Twist can be helpful for Pitta dosha people.

The Kapha dosha people use dynamic flow, such as Sun Salutations or Warrior Poses, to improve their metabolism.

Proper food consumption and herbal treatment provide all-around harmony for a healthy life.

A Harmony Journey: Story in Brief

Anjali was a corporate finance professional in her mid-thirties who always felt overwhelmed by work demands. She suffered from anxiety, faulty digestion, and sleepless nights. To seek refuge, she found solace in Ayurveda and Yoga.

Her Ayurvedic doctor identified her as Pitta-dominant with a Vata imbalance due to her erratic lifestyle. Anjali's healing journey began with a customized plan that included cooling pranayama practices like Sheetali and grounding yoga poses like Child's Pose and Cobra Pose. Along with a Pitta-balancing diet, she practiced daily Abhyanga followed by short, focused Yoga sessions.

Within weeks, she realized a change had occurred. Her anxiety diminished, her digestion improved, and she slept better. This harmonious blend of Ayurveda and Yoga brought her body back to normal and helped her achieve clarity of mind and emotional balance. She continues this practice today, feeling closer to herself and the world.

Conclusion

In short, the synergy of Yoga and Ayurveda has given us the ageless blueprint for life. As Ayurveda lays down the fundamental structure to learning about the body's requirements, the actual practice that needs to be performed to fulfill them is learned from Yoga. Therefore, taken as a whole, we can attain our poise, vigor, and mental balance in the best way possible for all of life. We become the natural rhythm through these ancient sciences and live in the rhythm of nature, alive and peaceful inside.

Chapter 27: Conclusion – Bringing it All Together

Ayurveda is more than a system of medicine; it is a way of life. It connects one with the rhythms of nature, regulates inner balance, and is in harmony with the body, mind, and spirit. This is brought through the book, which unfolds its concepts, therapies, and herbs, guiding us to health and living. We take the core concept of Ayurveda and then interweave practical tips on how to live a life that uses the teachings and practices of Ayurveda.

Summary of Ayurvedic Principles and Practices

- Understanding Your Prakriti (Constitution)

The Ayurvedic approach to health is based on understanding the vital balance of Vata, Pitta, and Kapha Doshas. Knowledge of one's constitution is the basis for wise diet, lifestyle, and daily self-care decisions.

- Agni (Digestive Fire):

Agni is central to Ayurveda, representing the metabolic and digestive functions. A strong Agni leads to health, while its imbalance causes disease. Following dietary guidelines, eating seasonal foods, and avoiding incompatible food combinations nurture Agni.

- Dinacharya and Ritucharya:

In Ayurveda, humans can reside on the waves of nature through daily and seasonal regimens. By following daily regimens, such as taking a massage oil bath in the morning and changing seasons, no one has ever been confronted by the illness of an imbalance.

- Panchakarma Therapies:

Vaman, Virechan, Basti, Nasya, and Leech Therapy are detoxifying therapies. They cleanse the body of toxins, stabilize doshas or humors, and infuse the mind and body with fresh life.

- Herbal Remedies:

Ayurvedic treatment relies on herbal remedies, including powders, decoctions, pastes, and oils. Herbs are a treasure box of holistic curative medicines that can treat several illnesses.

- Mind-Body Connection:

Shirodhara and Nasya's practices make one mentally lucid and emotionally sound. According to Ayurveda, the mind decides between health and disease.

- Yoga and Pranayama:

Ayurveda philosophy complements yoga and breathwork, promoting inner stability and enhancing energy. It brings harmony to the mind and body.

Ayurveda in Daily Life-Wake Up to a Great Day!

Begin every morning with tongue scraping, oil swishing, and drinking warm water. These will activate your digestive fire and detoxify you.

Eat what agrees with your dosha: Eat according to your Prakriti. Be present, and eat against your dosha imbalances. Eat freshly cooked, warm, nourishing foods without processed or incompatible foods.

- Get a Routine:

Ayurveda is all about routine and synchronizing body and mind, including food, sleep, and exercise.

- Incorporate Herbs:

Take turmeric, ginger, and Triphala regularly to maintain the proper digestion system, immunity power, and detoxification.

- Mindfulness Techniques

Perform yoga, meditation, and pranayama to control the body's stress and emotional balance.

- Listen to your Body

Listen to the early warning signs of disease—indigestion, overwhelm, weakness, or irritation—and shift your lifestyle and diet accordingly.

- Seasonal Balancing

A person's diet and lifestyle change with the seasons. For example, one may eat more extraordinary foods in summer and warmer foods in the winter.

Balance and Harmony in Lifestyle:

Health is not a destination but a journey. A healthy life happens when one is in sync with the harmony of nature and not attuned to one's body's wants. Consistent, simple steps like developing a morning routine or cultivating gratitude can lead to significant transformations over time, whether through appropriate diets or other healthy practices.

Let Ayurveda light up your path. It is an ancient science that meets a modern need. Open your heart and go for a walk on the earth.

Let these words of wisdom by Sage Charak guide you as we conclude this journey: "The understanding of a total nature of a thing does not arise from a fragmentary knowledge of it." Live harmoniously with Ayurveda to illuminate your life with the perfect understanding for a calm, serene, and balanced life for yourself.

Verses Kindler Publication

Verses Kindler Publication

Reach us through our website -

https://www.verseskindlerpublication.com/

For more information visit our Instagram or Facebook page.